Stone Benches

Understanding the Invisible Footprints of Dementia

By Judith Ingalsbe

Stone Benches Understanding the Invisible Footprints of Dementia

Stone Benches Understanding the Invisible Footprints of Dementia

Health & Fitness / Diseases / Alzheimer's & Dementia

E-book Version: Kindle

ISBN-13: 978-0692646229 (Symphony Publishing)

ISBN-10: 0692646221

Dedicated to my parents,
and to all those living with dementia.

And to the footprints who journey beside them.

"Now to him who is able to do immeasurably more than all
we ask or imagine,
according to His power that is at work within us."

Ephesians 3:20

My heartfelt thanks to:

My husband, Doug,
for your love, understanding, and support
as we continue to face the challenges of this disease.
Thank you for encouraging me to share these experiences
with others.

My daughters, Britta, Kristen, and Sierra
for loving your grandparents well through the
heartache and changes.
They would be proud of the beautiful women you are.

To all those who provided care for my parents
with compassion and dedication over the years.
A special thanks to Tammy, who has faithfully
accompanied me on this journey from beginning to end.

To Angie Steedman with Angie Steedman Photography for
her generous dedication of time and expertise of capturing our
loved ones so we can show the world #TheyHaveAName.

My good friend Lauri Williams for her commitment to me and
this book. I couldn't have done it without you.

To all those who believed in me, prayed for me,
and encouraged me to share this story.

Even When It Hurts by Joel Houston

Take this fainted heart
Take these tainted hands
Wash me in Your love
Come like grace again

Even when my strength is lost
I'll praise You
Even when I have no song
I'll praise You

Even when it's hard to find the words
Louder then I'll sing Your praise
I will only sing Your praise

Take this mountain weight
Take these ocean tears
Hold me through the trial
Come like hope again

Even when the fight seems lost
I'll praise You
Even when it hurts like hell
I'll praise You

Even when it makes no sense to sing
Louder then I'll sing Your praise
I will only sing Your praise
And my heart burns only for You
You are all - You are all I want
And my soul waits only for You
And I will sing till the morning has come

I will only sing Your praise

Even when the morning comes
I'll praise You
Even when the fight is won
I'll praise You

Even when my time on earth is done
Louder then I'll sing your praise
I will only sing Your praise

I will only sing Your praise
I will only sing Your praise
I will only sing Your praise

And my heart burns only for You
You are all You are all I want
And my soul waits only for You

6

And I will sing till the morning has come

Lord my heart burns only for You
You are all You are all I want
And my soul waits only for You
And I will sing till the miracle comes

I will only sing Your praise
I will only sing Your praise
I will only sing Your praise

Even when the morning comes
I'll praise You
Even when the fight is won
I'll praise You

Even when my time on earth is done
Louder then I'll sing your praise
I will only sing Your praise

Foreword: Husband of a Caregiver

by: Doug Ingalsbe

You are about to embark on a journey. A journey
without a clear beginning, a middle as murky as the
Mississippi River, and an end which leaves you longing
for just one more day with that person you knew. The
journey is Alzheimer's disease. The patient and their
loved ones are on this journey together. They are bound
by a disease that will strip them of recognition, force them
into rediscovery, and leave them searching for hope. A
hope that there will be a better tomorrow. A hope that
they will be able to swim to shore and find dry land. A
hope that there will be a peaceful and dignified end. A
hope that one day, no one will ever have to embark on the
same dreadful journey.

According to a 2015 Alzheimer's Association report,
there are an estimated 5.3 million Americans suffering
from this disease. A disease which has no clear
beginning. Forgotten conversations, inability to
remember a name or two, misplaced objects around the
house. It happens slowly. It seems innocent enough. We
all forget things from time to time, don't we?
Unfortunately, for the patient of early Alzheimer's

disease, things will not get better. The disease starts to eat at the brain. Scientists know exactly what is happening. Through years of research they can tell us why this journey is beginning. Sadly, they can't do anything about it.

Your journey starts to take you down a mysterious, painful, and troublesome path. Your loved one doesn't know you, they don't know the friends who come to visit, and they can no longer do the job that provided for you and your family. They can't dress themselves, they can't feed themselves, they can't bathe without your help, and they can't even tell you "thank you for taking care of me". You are paddling through that muddy river in a current so swift that every day you feel like the battle is being lost. You are spending every ounce of energy in your body and resources in your bank account hoping to find the dry land that seems to be getting farther and farther away.

This book will take you on that journey. Page by page, you will find you are not alone. You are 5.3 million strong. You will read about the very personal, sad, comical, and joyful journey we have been on with you. You will find the hope you are searching for. You will find peace in knowing you can start over every day. You will not be ashamed or afraid of what you are doing, not doing, or want to do over again.

OUR hope is that through reading about our journey you will embrace every day of this awful disease with courage, passion, and pride. Courage to face what you must, passion to be patient with your care, and pride in knowing you are doing a thankless job. By the end of your journey you will be at peace, as will the person you are committed to caring for.

Chapters

Introduction

Everything is in the process of being forgotten,
but who we are and who we have been remains forever.

Most will not read this book out of mere curiosity, nor did I write it by accident. Tragically, it is likely someone we love has been struck with one of the horrific diseases classified as dementia. Alzheimer's is the most common, a disease which attacks and deteriorates the brain. One day our loved one was living life to its fullest, then subtle changes occurred, concerns arose, a diagnosis was made, and their life, as well as ours, would never be the same.

Those of us walking this path understand the person we once knew has been inexplicably changed forever. We miss who our loved ones were and are saddened by what they can no longer do. We have researched, sought answers, worried about the future, grieved the past, and forged into the unknown. Sorrow, guilt, fear, anger, and an overwhelming sense of loss are the familiar emotions of this horrible disease. Because of our shared challenges and heartache, we have become kindred spirits.

You may be curious about the disease because of behaviors you are just beginning to notice in your loved one. Perhaps they have recently been diagnosed, or you may be like me and have lived this reality for many years.

12

Whatever the case, this is our common walk, wherever we might be on the journey. For those who have received a diagnosis, we recall the details of that day as if it were yesterday. The tragedy is etched in our minds, an unforgettable horror. From the day this becomes our reality, we navigate the physical, medical, and financial decisions for our loved one's care.

It is very likely you are looking for answers, hope, or the encouragement needed to make it through another day. You may be so exhausted from this disease consuming your every thought and demanding every ounce of energy, the last thing you want to do is read a book on the subject. I understand. I have been there in the moments of desperation, as well as pure frustration. Let me assure you, we do not have to merely endure this disease. There are beautiful moments waiting to be discovered on a daily basis when we learn to live, despite this affliction, in the presence of our loved one.

If you are looking for someone who holds all the answers, this book is not for you. I have made more than my fair share of mistakes and continue to learn on a daily basis. This is my wish for you as well. My mission is to inspire you to get involved and join efforts to find a cure. I hope to encourage you to educate yourself about the disease and become an advocate for those affected. If you are reading this book ten years from now, please know things have changed since I shared these insights. Medications, treatment, and our understanding of this illness are constantly developing.

Other things, however, will never change. Your loved one's need for your dependable love, as well as a voice for them, will remain constant. Their need to be understood is eternal. If this is not possible in every situation, at the very least, insure they are respected and enjoyed. Enter their world, laugh with them, and continue to enjoy a life rich with adventure. They will greatly benefit from your consistent and enlightened care. I promise, you will be pleasantly surprised by how much they have to offer. There is a joy that is undeniably experienced when we join these folks where they exist.

This is the story of a family, much like yours, who found ourselves staring this terrible disease in the face. We can run, but we cannot hide, from the painful reality of this tragedy. We do not, however, have to live in frustration and hopelessness. Yes, this is a story of a terrible disease with heartbreaking consequences. However, despite the inevitable obstacles we face, there is

14

potential for a fulfilled life rich with dignity and enjoyment for our loved ones. Let the tears, as well as the laughter, wash over you. Gather refreshment which you can, in turn, offer your loved one. Be encouraged-the gift of time, however long, is ours to enjoy!

"Because I have a name, remember I am still the person you know and love."

Footprints

The beautiful imprint of who we have become
and that which we aspire to be.

Over a decade ago, my beautiful Aunt June quietly and willingly took on the role of surrogate mother to me after my own mom was diagnosed with Alzheimer's disease. Honestly, I had not even realized she stepped into this position, now walking beside me in the footprints where Mom's once were, until many years later. Of course, I acknowledged her support and dedication right away. She was just a phone call away, or in reality a few blocks drive, when I needed encouragement.

By the time my fortieth birthday rolled around, my mother did not remember my name, much less my birthday. This would have absolutely devastated her to know. She made my celebrations special, without fail, on a yearly basis. I put on a strong front, but if the truth be known, it was crushing. Remarkably, Aunt June and Uncle Bill, Mom's brother, took me out to celebrate my birthday on my special day that year. Since then, not a year has passed without this special couple showering me with grand attention. It is impossible that they understand what this has meant to me.

Although no one could ever replace my beautiful mother, my aunt certainly filled those empty footprints well. This void would have been devastating without her presence and consistent love in my life. She has always been special to me, but this past decade our relationship has grown into so much more. Although she still manages quite well in her own home, Aunt June now needs a little assistance occasionally. Always grateful for any little thing we do for her, she goes out of her way to thank us. If she only knew what she had done for me.

Aunt June now carries a security device which will allow her to call for help if she falls or finds herself in a perilous situation. If I am not able to reach her for a period of time, I often get concerned about her well-being. Fortunately, I can simply glance at an app on my phone, which will readily inform me of her precise location. "Oh, of course," I will say to my husband, "I forgot she had a hair appointment today." Some may view this as a terrible invasion of privacy, but she assures me it gives her a peace of mind. My aunt will even ask me, "Did you notice I went to the market today?"

Admittedly, this type of monitoring has the potential to be rather unnerving, especially when one is not aware they are being tracked. When my youngest daughter was in college, she had the wonderful opportunity to study abroad. As a result, she enjoyed one glorious summer of memory making, and studying I presume, in London. Before she left, she found an app, which we both downloaded to our phones. This allowed us to communicate through a messaging system. It worked beautifully.

The opportunity to stay in contact with her in this way was priceless. It is amazing how a quick sentence during the day gives one a feeling of being connected. One day I received a welcomed message from my daughter. "Are you going out for lunch today?" Ironically, I was dining at a restaurant with Aunt June when I received her message. I did not remember telling her my plans for the day, but then she did know my routine rather well.

My next stop, after kissing my beautiful aunt goodbye, was the chiropractor. As I waited to receive my much anticipated adjustment, the following message appeared on my phone: "Going to Dr. Collier today?" How did she know? She was full of lucky guesses. I would now be heading home, after a quick, unexpected stop by a friend's house to pick up some strawberries fresh from her garden. She phoned me while I was at the chiropractor and I was delighted to accept her offer. As

I began to pull out of my friend's driveway, this unnerving message arrived: "Tell Miss Lisa I said hello!"

My next response was direct and straightforward, "*What is going on?*" Apparently, yet not surprisingly, unbeknownst to me the app we were using also had the capacity to track the movements of the device on which it was installed. Thankfully, I was not in the habit of frequenting questionable places. I took a moment to silently acknowledge my gratefulness for leading a quiet, predictable life.

Arriving home, I received this message on my phone: "So funny, it looks like you parked in the water!" The app was not as precise as one might think. Having missed my location by several hundred yards, it mistakenly placed me in the middle of a neighborhood pond. It was curious to me that this location device was only functioning on one end of this two-way street. I found it unfortunate that I was not privy to my daughter's visits to Buckingham Palace to have tea with the Queen.

We are preoccupied with knowing where others, as well as ourselves, have been. Many a concerned parent has installed tracking devices on their teenager's car. My three daughters will be relieved to know the level of trust they earned prohibited me from ever considering such a measure. That being said, unfortunately, I did not have the same level of trust in our four legged friends. Both of our precious canines are equipped with chips. These will alert anyone who scans their furry necks to the location of their responsible owners.

There are devices in place to track our every move. Credit card chips notify anyone having access to our account of our exact location, as we swipe our way through town. Most stores will be able to tell us the precise date and time we shopped there, as well as what we bought. If we lose our keys along the way, a tracking device can locate them for us. Not only are we interested in knowing where we have been, it is also becoming increasingly imperative to know how many steps the journey has taken us.

I freely admit, nothing is more frustrating than spending an extra ten minutes on the Elliptical, purposely parking at the far end of parking lots throughout the day, and taking the stairs instead an elevator, only to discover the Fitbit was absentmindedly left behind. If a trip to the mall was involved, the day is all but ruined. Those of you with Fitbits cannot even pretend you do not know what I am talking about.

It is no longer enough to simply remember events of our lives. We must document them with exacting preciseness. It is curious how keenly important this is to us. Why are we so obsessed with the past? I believe it is because we are, unfortunately, inclined to place the value of who we are in where we have been and what we have done. Our worth is often found in the imprint of the footprints of our past.

Additionally, the successes, as well as the mistakes, are documented to serve as guides for the future. If we failed to walk far enough today, we will do better tomorrow. At the end of the week we receive the summary of our performance. Our worth can then be appraised on this valuable information. Knowing where we have been and how well we have traveled that journey is immensely important to us. There is yet another reason we are interested in where we have been. It is in these footprints we also find precious memories.

Footprints hold valuable information of who we know, what we have done, as well as priceless stories of the past. Without this information, we would be unable to function. Absent of these recollections, our future moves would become difficult at best, although likely impossible. Our next step is based upon the knowledge we have of the outcomes of past performances. Just as a comedian will cease telling a joke past audiences did not respond well to, hopefully, we will not continue to make decisions which failed to provide a positive outcome.

When I was six weeks old, my family packed up and moved from my parents' hometown to a nearby city. My father's family owned and operated an auto dealership in their small town. The business was started by my grandfather with just a few cars and had proven successful for many years. Times were changing and these small town car dealers were finding it difficult to keep up with big city car lots. The business was ultimately sold, which resulted in my dad being out of a job. With a new baby and nine-year-old son, a move to the larger city with more opportunities was imperative.

Dad eventually found work and my family settled into a quiet suburb, which is now located in the center of our ever-growing city. Once I started school, I walked to the bus stop each morning, which was located down the street. On the rare occasion it snowed, I had the distinct honor of following my brother's footprints through the snow swept yards. By now, he was in high school with much longer strides than those of his six-year-old sister. I

22

distinctly remember leaping to the next large imprint left on the soft, snowy ground.

After a few misplaced steps of the past had resulted in treacherous travels through large snow drifts, I learned it was in my best interest to follow the true and proven steps of my beloved brother. Most of the time I was quite successful, at other times, despite my best efforts, my leap was disappointedly short. This would result in my pants being covered with a dusting of snow. However, I was usually able to put my best foot forward, having devised a plan based on the knowledge I had acquired.

It is not just the experiences of others who have gone before us on which we gauge our future steps. The results we have achieved from our experiences are also examined. We remember, take note, and duly adjust our next step. Great value is placed on how well we process the past and successfully direct the future. We take great pride in the recognition received from our achievements. I suppose it has always been this way, whether the goal be to build a fortress strong enough to protect against the impending armies or successfully capture wild game for dinner on the frontier.

Eventually, my dad found success in a career selling investments in the city. He was a hardworking man, rising before dawn and often arriving home well after dark. The prize for this commitment, besides the ability to put food on the table for his family, was at times the rare opportunity to earn a company incentive-a trip to an impressive location. When I was seven, my dad earned such a trip to Acapulco.

To my delight, he announced we would all be joining him on this vacation. I was eager to miss a week of school to experience a faraway place with my family. This was to be my first glimpse of the majestic ocean, which began my lifetime fondness. The sound of the waves, smell of the salt, everything about the ocean filled me in a unique and wonderful way. It was delightful to experience the water splashing onto my feet as the sand shifted between my toes. I was fascinated.

Every possible moment was spent playing on the beach and splashing in the waves. My favorite recollection is riding on Dad's shoulders as he ran through the sand and into the ocean. The waves lapped up onto my legs as we went deeper and deeper into the beautiful blue water. Other children splashed in the waves as families enjoyed the beautiful setting. Some days we floated for what seemed like hours in the waves.

One day Dad and I ventured farther than we had been before. Looking back, I realize there was not the usual activity in the water. At the time, we hardly took note. We were lost in the delight of the ocean, oblivious to anything or anyone else. I was captivated by its immensity. Looking out over the horizon, the possibilities seemed endless. It was one of the most majestic, peaceful feelings I had ever known.

In contrast, from the shore, Mom suddenly became concerned at the commotion on the beach. She watched in horror as voices frantically warned two lone swimmers to return. The language was unfamiliar, but the message was clear, there was danger in the water. Eventually, Dad and I realized something was terribly wrong. I have vivid memories of my mom in the distance desperately waving her arms in the air.

By this time a crowd had gathered on the beach, as the beautiful ocean was transformed into a ghastly horror right before their eyes. It was not until we reached the shore that our attention was directed to sharks circling in the area we had been only moments before. Despite this frightful experience, my family and I made beautiful memories on that trip. My love for the ocean continued to grow and visiting the beach remained one of my Dad's greatest joys.

When my own three daughters experienced the ocean for the first time, his was the hand they would hold. While visiting Disneyworld, an impulsive day trip from our well planned vacation landed us on a beautiful beach with not another soul in sight. Three tiny sets of footprints decorated the beach in Florida, alongside the larger prints of their beloved leader. Our afternoon was spent picnicking and building sand castles. Dad and the girls splashed in the water and walked the beach collecting seashells. Mom and I spent precious moments under the umbrella, soaking up one of the most beautiful days I have ever known.

Many years later it would be my footprints next to Dad's as we made his final walk along a beach together in California. The ocean's familiarity drew me back after my mom lost her battle with Alzheimer's disease. Dad and I packed our bags and made plans to visit his sister on the coast. My Auntie planned our week-the only agenda being to sit beside the ocean. Our grieving hearts were comforted by the beautiful sights and calming sounds. We had the amazing experience of visiting a different beach each day.

While recently sifting through some of my parents' belongings I discovered a large white bucket of seashells. This find brought back memories of visits to my parents' winter retreat on The Gulf in their retirement years. After every morning walk, Dad emptied his pockets to reveal a treasured find: a few small, beautiful shells worthy of his notice. Apparently, these shells, collected over many years, had gained a place of importance in my parents' lives.

They were among the treasures of a carefully packed box. Yearbooks, photos, a family Bible, awards, their marriage certificate, these shells, had apparently been deemed as their most precious possessions. Most would view the shells as ordinary, as they are similar in color and size, absent of the slightest hint of extraordinary. To my dad, however, they were remarkable.

These gems, exceptional enough to interrupt a walk, had persuaded him to stop, bend down, and successfully grasp the prize before an impending wave swept it away. Time and again he repeated this process. After careful analyzation, he determined which to keep. After many years a considerable collection was gathered.

Each precious shell he chose would become a welcome decoration for their winter retreat. When it was time to leave, these tiny treasures were not cast aside, but rather packed alongside belongings to accompany them home. Ultimately, these remarkable keepsakes were chosen to inhabit a box of heirlooms. Each was irreplaceable, representing a walk along the shore, never to be repeated.

Picture life as a journey, as we follow the footprints laid out in front of us. We can't see too far in the horizon-the path is barely visible beyond the next turn. So we keep our eyes focused on the next move, as we follow the footsteps ahead of us. If we lose focus, we eventually realize we are off-course and quickly take the steps necessary to regain our direction. Treasures are carefully collected, our precious memories, along the way.

This is our reality-life as we know it. We make sense of our days by the value placed on our ability to maintain direction as we make progress towards the goal. Respect, self-worth, and dignity are all the result of a journey well-traveled. Sometimes steady, at other times faltering, but always able to pick up our foot and place it on the next step ahead of us. We can look back, as well, and see what lies behind us-the memories, the achievements, the mistakes. These are an imprint of who we have become, and what we aspire to be. They serve as guides for decisions of the future. Everything we have ever known, everyone we hold dear, is found in these footprints.

Imagine what would happen if they could no longer be found. What if waves washed over the visible footprints, rendering them obliterated? The past erased, our direction no longer visible, and our precious memories, treasured over time, swept back into the sea. What if reality as we know it was wiped out, wave by crashing wave? Adversity circled, and our family was struck.

This is how it must be for those with dementia, the waves of confusion washing over the footprints ahead, erasing the next viable thought. Carefully collected memories tossed into the water, never to be retrieved again. What would it be like to live in the reality of this existence, with nothing by which to gauge the next move or remember the realities of the past?

Join me as we learn to walk along the treacherous shores of this disease. Despite inevitable devastation lurking in the water, there is hope and encouragement awaiting. As the keepers and facilitators of memories, we will learn to gather precious treasures alongside the invisible footprints of dementia. There is still much beauty awaiting our discovery!

"Because I have a name, please continue to treasure the memories we make together."

The Journey
Understanding the path before us
as we learn to walk these unchosen steps.

Make no mistake, this disease is a long and treacherous journey. Since it is very likely the process will be a long-term proposition, it is in our best interest to invest some effort in learning as much as we can about the disease. Alzheimer's is the most common form of dementia. It is a progressive disease which interferes with a person's ability to function. According to the latest statistics, one in three people over the age of eighty have some form of dementia.

Although dementia is widely viewed as a memory problem, in reality, everything the brain controls is eventually affected. Given the fact our brains control virtually everything in our being, this obviously has far reaching effects. Deterioration of the brain is not a normal part of aging, nor is it a mental illness. It is, however, a long, heartbreaking death as the disease steals abilities and functions one by one. Until a cure is found, it will remain irreversibly progressive and terminal.

In the early stages of the disease, signs are often subtle and easy to misinterpret. We may reason our loved one is depressed, or perhaps stress is causing them to make more mistakes than usual. After all, we all can be forgetful at times. Knowing the signs and differences between normal, occasional lapses in memory and the onset of the disease is crucial. A doctor will not be able to pick up on these slight changes in a regular visit. It is up to us, as loved ones, to identify warning signs as they are observed in everyday life.

It is still unknown what causes this disease, although two categories of genes have been linked to its occurrence. One specific gene has been associated with an inherited risk factor. According to the Alzheimer's Association, although a family presence of the disease can increase the risk, having both parents with the disease only bears a slightly higher risk than that of a person with little or no family history of the disease.

According to the latest statistics, five point three million Americans have been diagnosed with this disease; that is one in ten people over the age of sixty-five. Unfortunately, by the time you read these statistics, they will no longer be accurate. Someone in the United States alone develops Alzheimer's every sixty-seven seconds. It is estimated by 2050 as many as sixteen million of us will have been handed this terrible news.

Despite the immensity of the disease, caring for a loved one with Alzheimer's, or other memory impairment, is a very personal act of loving dedication. The process will require commitment, as well as a heaping dose of understanding. Alzheimer's disease is the fourth leading cause of death among the elderly. However, the aged are not the only group at risk.

Early-onset Alzheimer's, or the occurrence of the disease in those under the age of sixty-five, represents five percent of all people affected. Additionally, this disease is responsible for taking the lives of more women than breast cancer and ovarian cancer combined. Two-thirds of those with Alzheimer's are women, simply because they tend to live longer.

Those inflicted have done nothing to cause this condition, but will suffer the effects for many years. As we learn more about the condition of dementia, we can help our loved ones have a more productive and enjoyable life. Before we can effectively walk alongside them, we must first have an understanding of how this disease affects the brain. The information presented here is not intended as medical advice, but rather as insight equipping us to pursue the best quality of life for those we love.

Dementia is an umbrella term comprised of numerous cognitive loss conditions. There are many causes for dementia, and many specific diseases falling under this classification. According to the Mayo Clinic, some dementias, such as Alzheimer's disease, occur on their own, not as a result of another disease. Others are the result of another disease or injury to the brain. Dementias can be classified in a variety of ways and are often grouped together by what they have in common, such as what part of the brain is affected, or whether they worsen with time.

Dementias which cause a patient's mental capacity to decline over time are known as progressive dementias. Alzheimer's would be an example of a progressive dementia, following a predictable course. Other dementias, such as those caused by a reaction to medications or an infection, may be reversible with treatment. Our loved ones deserve our dedication in seeking answers which will affect their future. This is why it is imperative to find a doctor who will take the time to fully explore the symptoms and order the appropriate testing to exhaust all other possibilities before making a diagnosis.

Unfortunately, the majority of dementias are progressive, worsening in time. There are several main types of these progressive dementias. Regardless of how the dementia manifests itself, there are similarities, the primary one being the predictive deterioration of the brain over time. There are literally hundreds of dementias, most being treated with identical medications. (See appendix for a list of common dementias.)

The brain consists of billions of cells, each with a special task. Everything we do starts with a signal from the brain. Thinking, learning, and memory are controlled by the brain, as are seeing, breathing, and movement. Alzheimer's disease prevents the cells from functioning as they should. Eventually the cells die and will no longer send any messages at all.

Current research is being directed at understanding these connections. I recently attended a lecture outlining studies which are focused on forming new neural cells and pathways in the brain. Dr. Sandra Petersen, associate professor at The University of Texas at Tyler, explained new research strongly suggests the brain is capable of making these connections with certain stimuli.

This enables people with memory impairment to reconnect with old memories and build new ones.

Although scientists have been studying this principal for over a century, breakthroughs in the area of neuroplasticity are fairly recent. The theory disputes the longstanding idea that our brain is incapable of developing new brain cells. Within the last twenty years, studies have revolutionized this belief. Neuroplasticity maintains the brain's plastic-like ability to self-mend and flexibly adapt as needed by forming new neural cells and pathways.

This research is significant, especially given the fact changes may begin in the brain twenty years or more before diagnosis of Alzheimer's disease is made. This is long before current tests can detect the disease. Once scientists have a better understanding of the brain's capability to mend, the diseases of dementia can potentially be treated much earlier, long before symptoms are present.

For the estimated forty-four million people in the world currently affected by Alzheimer's disease alone, this is very good news. The statistics are staggering; however, the heart of the tragedy lives within the loved one we care for. The reality for them is the area of their brain involved in thinking, planning, and remembering is damaged. Outward signs begin occurring when plaques and tangles spread to areas affecting speech and understanding. Tragically, those affected will soon not be able to care for themselves.

Almost twenty years ago, I drove to my parents' house, picked up my mom, and brought her to my home. If only I could turn back time, erase the heartache, what I would give. We were facing a terrible tragedy; I needed and wanted Mom with me. Perhaps I could engage her in an activity, something enjoyable to get our minds off the horrible reality. All Mom wanted to do, could do, was sit on the sofa, gazing out the window, in the privacy of her own tears.

I frequently sat with her, suggesting alternatives, anything at all to release her mind from this anguish she was experiencing. She continued to silently look out the window, quietly sobbing, unable to respond. My mother was gone, absent from the reality of the present. If I could have taken her pain, a heartache which to this day I cannot comprehend, I would have. All I could do for my mom was be present and offer my support, as I watched my mother's heart slowly die.

My grief was raw as well, but I freely acknowledge it was nothing compared to my mother's. For although my presence could be beside her as a daughter, her son was gone. When my brother was forty-two years old, he was tragically murdered. His story is far too immense to be contained within these pages, but what I can tell you is my mother was never the same after that day. His horrific death took a piece of her that never returned. Although her diagnosis would not come until several years later, her absence was felt immediately.

Mom sank into a deep depression after losing her son. I have often wondered if her mind simply could not comprehend the tragedy and freely relinquished itself to depression, and eventually Alzheimer's disease. When I imagine her heartache and the incomprehensible pain she was experiencing, it seems reasonable to me an escape from reality would be preferable. Yet I was grieving as well, which I am quite certain clouds my interpretation of this season of our lives. I offer all of you who have lost a child, some of my dearest friends and strangers alike, a prayer for healing and peace.

What I do know is our family was on autopilot for a few years as we attempted to seek a new normal. My dad dealt with his grief by submerging himself in work, as well as his second occupation by now of travel. He planned wonderful trips for my mom and himself. It is just now occurring to me his tactic of distraction was similar to mine, only on a much grander scale. The heartbreaking reality is: if a thousand pictures of our lives were tossed on the ground, I could sort with certainty if they were taken previous to or after this tragedy.

There was an invisible line drawn the day we were notified of my brother's murder, the day I brought my grieving mother to my home. She was never the same. By simply looking into the eyes of my mother in a thousand pictures, I could easily identify the timeframe they were taken. There is absolutely no basis for what I am about to say, except the observations of a daughter. I believe my mom was vulnerable, because of her weakened emotional state, to this disease. What I do know with certainty is I lost my mom that day.

In reality, her brain could have already been experiencing changes due to this disease. Researchers now believe these changes may occur many years before any outward signs are apparent. Scientists believe shrinkage in the hippocampus, an area of the outer layer of the brain, or cortex, is especially severe in a brain diseased by Alzheimer's. The hippocampus is key in the brain's ability to form new memories. By the time the disease has reached the severe stage, the brain has shrunk dramatically and is severely damaged due to widespread cell death.

There are two key components researchers believe contribute to this disease, plaques and tangles. As we age, most people develop plaques, or deposits of protein fragments. Just as plaque deposits in veins and arteries affect the efficiency of the heart, their presence in the brain inhibits it from working properly. Those affected with Alzheimer's disease tend to develop much more plaque than those unaffected.

In addition, other proteins create twisted fibers, called tangles. These interfere with signals being sent from the brain. Plaques and tangles typically begin in the area of the brain involved with memory and spread to other areas. Eventually, every area of the brain, and therefore every aspect of the person's function, is affected. The average life expectancy, after signs are apparent in those with Alzheimer's, is approximately eight to ten years.

Unfortunately, I have witnessed firsthand the heartbreak of this horrible disease. This terrible tragedy has been devastating our family for over thirty years. I am eager for some good news. It is long overdue. This is why when I hear about hopeful research, I want to shout it from the rooftop! Despite the incredible length of this journey, I am still seeking information and finding valuable insight I can apply to our situation. Last week, the lecture I attended left me feeling hopeful and extremely encouraged.

The speaker shared the results of the twelve week study she conducted last year with a $30,000 grant from Baylor Health Care. The results were impressive. In a brain diseased by Alzheimer's, it was once thought impossible to build brain cells by stimulating or training the brain. This study, involving the use of PARO robots for treating Alzheimer's disease and other forms of dementia, is the first of its kind in the United States.

Sixty patients, treated individually or in small groups, participated in the study. They were prescribed twenty minute treatments, involving interaction with the PARO, three times a week. Pulse rate, skin response, as well as oxygen saturation, which measures stress, were documented. The goal was to decrease anxiety and depression in patients, as well as their reliance on prescription drugs. This doctor now routinely prescribes this treatment to her patients in lieu of certain medications. The treatment? An adorable robotic seal.

Dr. Takanori Shibata, a Japanese scientist, invented the PARO robotic. These robots, programmed specifically for patients with dementia, are designed to treat anxiety and depression, common side effects of the disease. The furry white animal with large blinking eyes mimics a real baby seal and is designed to evoke a nurturing response in patients with dementia. I freely admit seals have always been my most beloved animal at the zoo, but I say with the utmost impartiality, these guys are cute!

I had the opportunity to hold this robotic baby seal, which is programmed to respond to voice and touch, as well as the individual's personality. The adorable robot's personality is developed over time, much like our furry friends respond to us dependent on our interactions in the past. There was something unexplainably captivating about this experience. Every person in the room, men and women alike, were enthralled with this animal. I can hardly imagine having the opportunity to spend twenty minutes connecting with her.

Make no mistake, although this creature is instantly calming and captivating, (we all were more than curious how she would respond to our various interactions) this revolutionary development does more than mitigate boredom in dementia patients. Petersen's research found a thirty percent overall decrease in the amount of as-needed medications given to control anxiety. Since many common disruptive behaviors of dementia patients stem from anxious uncertainty, these findings have the potential for monumental, far reaching effects.

Considering the average dementia patient takes fourteen to thirty pills per day, translating to a cost of at least $800 to $1,200 a month, the finding is enormously significant. Although my loved ones' conservative doctor prescribed far less medication, I can attest to the staggering cost of dementia related prescriptions and the financial impact it has made on my family. Additionally, Petersen's study could provide the strong scientific evidence needed to result in Medicare covering the cost of robotic pet medical treatments in the future.

The health risks alone, including organ failure, resulting from the elderly consuming this enormous amount of medication, demands that our attention be directed to studies, such as this. Quality of life for those with dementia is already being positively affected on a small scale thanks to this study. Hopefully, this will soon become a mainstream dementia treatment. It is encouraging, to say the least.

"Because I have a name,
please learn all you can about this disease."

Under the Umbrella

Wrapped in the protection
found only in the safety of a mother's love.

One of the fondest memories I have of my mom is sitting on the floor by her chair as she stroked my hair. The protection, devotion, and love she exuded was almost tangible. Time seemed to stand still as her gentle fingers wove my windblown locks into symmetry. She made me feel safe, as only a mother could. I remember wishing I could stay there forever, under the umbrella of her love, hidden away from the world and its problems, from the realities of life.

Perhaps it was the unspoken sentiments we shared on these occasions, or the memories these feelings conjured up that made these moments so special. Even now, at times when I need strength to face the day, I shut my eyes and can feel this incredible gift, the incomparable love of my mom. Those moments were swiftly taken from me almost seven years ago, but this remains one of the most recent and treasured memories I have with her.

Long after this horrible disease stole my mom's ability to tell me how much I meant to her, she showered me with her presence in this way. This beautiful form of communication was rediscovered by accident. I was sitting on the floor by Mom's chair, sorting through pictures, when she instinctively reached out and touched my hair. Memories came flooding back of childhood moments sitting at her feet as she brushed my hair.

There are no words to adequately describe the feeling of being transported back in time by this simple gesture. All I can say is, at that moment, I was her precious little girl again and she was my mom. For an instant in time, I was shielded from all the decisions, heartache, and pain this disease had dealt us. Safe in the cocoon of my mother's love, I could simply experience this inexplicable peace.

I believe these moments afforded me a tangible glimpse of the past and the incredible gift it was to be this woman's daughter. Although this disease is a part of my mom's story, it does not define who she was. Alzheimer's was her companion for approximately one-eighth of her life, which left many decades of an existence lived free from its curse. If I am to tell the story of her journey with this disease, the essence of who she was before it became her companion must first be understood.

I recently attended the ninety-fifth birthday party of a dear friend in Mom's hometown. The guest of honor happened to be my parents' Sunday School teacher when they were newly married. I did not know most of the guests, but when they discovered who my mom was, her sweetness and generosity became the inevitable topic of conversation. Considering the number of women who have described the beautiful clothes Mom made for them, I am convinced a style show could be organized. This lovely woman had a way of making each person she met feel special.

When my parents married, Dad's sister, my dear Auntie, became the beneficiary of Mom's sewing talent. She remembers these dresses well and continues to credit them as being among the most beautiful pieces she has ever owned. The hostess of the birthday party, the guest of honor's niece, also described in great detail the clothing my mother sewed for her. Each piece Mom made was out of sheer generosity and adoration for the recipient.

Not only a talented seamstress, my mom was accomplished at all types of needlework as well. Her attention to detail, as well as her patience were admirable. I personally witnessed many instances of Mom taking out and reworking the tiniest error. I inadvertently challenged the extent of her fortitude the day she introduced me to a needlework sampler. With enormous patience she demonstrated the details of each stitch: popcorn, cross, running, satin. I listened intently, then took my project to the backyard with every intention of impressing my mother.

It was a beautiful spring afternoon. I can picture the exact spot where I was sitting on the red brick wall of my childhood home. I am quite sure I chose this location to be in the company of my new beloved pet: an adorable hen named D.D. Although I was eager to learn needlepoint, I was even more intent on being just like my talented mom. After a considerable portion of the sampler was complete and a substantial amount of time invested, I ran to the house to show Mom my beautiful handiwork. The look on her face was a delicate, clever balance of amusement and compassion.

The unfortunate reality is I had stitched the entire sampler to my skort. I should mention, for those of you not a product of the sixties, a skort is a combination of a skirt and shorts. These fashion forward beauties would surely have made a trendsetter out of me, had I not been ejected from my first grade class for wearing one, but that is another story. Suffice it to say, it was deemed to be too much short and not enough skirt. Apparently my skort was not only unwelcome in the classroom, but the front panel was a menace to needlework projects as well.

Knowing myself as well as I do, I am quite certain there were tears, bouts of exasperation, and possibly even a sampler adorned skort abandoned on the kitchen floor. However, pouting was simply not an option in the warmth of my mom's sunny disposition. Eventually there was a considerable amount of laughter. Ultimately, together Mom and I painfully took out every stitch and the project resumed. My childhood was filled with laughter. I recall Mom finding amusement in everyday moments, as well as situations others would regard stressful.

My family loved the occasional summer vacation to Colorado and the vast array of activities it provided. One summer we were horseback riding up the trails of a beautiful mountain. Dad led the way behind the guide, followed by my brother, and Mom, then I brought up the rear. We were on a steep incline when I began to ponder the reason my mom seemed to be rotating from one side of the horse to the other. I had no more determined that her saddle must be loose when it propelled upside down to the horse's belly, depositing my mother on the rocky trail.

It took Mom a moment to gain her composure as the guide helped her to her feet. I was horrified having witnessed Mom's horrific fall. Tears were flowing down her blushed and dusty cheeks; I know it must have hurt. She was not crying, however, but rather laughing uncontrollably at her unfortunate tumble. Both of my parents taught me to find humor in situations as we navigated the difficult circumstances of our lives.

Many years later, after I moved away to college, Mom and Dad welcomed a new boarder into their home. The woman credited with passing this joyful gene to Mom was facing one of the biggest crises of her life. My grandma was diagnosed with dementia when she was eighty-three years old. The family agreed to move her from the house where my grandparents raised their six children. Soon after, Mom and her siblings began the process of shutting down Grandma's little home of over forty years.

I called Mom often that fall to ask how the process was going. Her comical description of packing Grandma's dresser is my most vivid recollection of those conversations. She relayed to me, "I could hardly get one drawer put in a box before your grandma had another box unpacked and neatly stacked back in a drawer." Grandma's house held so many precious memories of holidays, summer visits, gardening, and playing in the washhouse. I could not imagine her living any other place. For all the memories I had, Grandma must have treasured a million more.

Eventually she settled into a life with my parents and Mom became her devoted caregiver. That Christmas I came home and eagerly joined Mom and Grandma in the kitchen for holiday baking. Grandma had made her infamous cream nut cake for more years than my life could document. This particular year, Mom baked the layers, we iced the cake, and Grandma and I were charged with the duty of decorating it with pecans.

As far as I know, there is just one pecan pattern worthy of such a cake. I am aware that, despite what transpired next, one might assume Grandma was somehow in the right. However, I know this for certain: in my vast observations of cream nut cake decorating, what I was attempting to achieve was Grandma's patented design. This would be a cinch, or piece of cake I should say. One by one, Grandma and I started placing the pecans.

Soon I discovered each pecan I put on the cake was removed by Grandma and haphazardly stuck in another position. I got Mom's attention, in hopes she would move Grandma to another task or, at the very least, talk some sense into her. I would like to think my patience and understanding of this disease have developed considerably since that day. My wise mother simply stated, "Let Grandma show you how to do it, Judy." Show me how to do it? Was my mother blind?

Mom was a patient, wise, and caring soul who had learned these qualities largely from her mom. I am quite certain my mother felt her wisdom was lost on me that day. I just remember feeling terribly frustrated with the whole situation. Not surprisingly, this moment is documented with a picture. As one might expect, Grandma looks quite determined and I appear to be laden with confusion. How thankful I am for the seeds of patience my mom planted in me. If our mothers only knew how their words take root in our souls and help mold us into more beautiful human beings.

Not only did my grandma pass down a legacy of wisdom and love, unfortunately, dementia was also prevalent in her family. My first encounter with this condition was when I was about seven. Grandma took me to the nursing home to visit her brother who clearly no longer remembered who she was. She was visibly shaken. I vividly recall her sentiments as we left, "I hope the good Lord takes me before I get in that condition." I assumed it was a rite of passage for the elderly to simply lose their memory. Thankfully, this is not the case.

It was, however, my grandma's fate. As it turned out, the good Lord blessed us with her sweet presence for ten years after she developed Alzheimer's. Eventually, she was moved to a neighborhood nursing home a few blocks from my parents' home. As I reflect on the care my grandma received over thirty years ago, I realize many things have changed for the better. This disease was even more of a mystery than it is today. The Alzheimer's Association was newly formed and trial drugs were just beginning to be developed.

The protocol for patient care was also vastly different. At the time, fall risks were tied to their chairs. After Grandma broke her hip, this was procedure for her. My mom could not bear the thought of her being strapped to a chair and was determined to find another way. She had soon designed embroidered vests for Grandma to wear which kept her from standing and abolished the need for straps. Mom's compassion was rewarded by the beautiful, contented lady in the beautifully adorned vests. Ten years afforded us many more memories with Grandma.

One of my favorites is of a snow storm with drifts so high it was impossible to get the car out of the garage. I knew Mom would be disappointed by not being able to get to Grandma's and feed her breakfast, as was her daily routine. "Oh, I am still planning to go," she said. Moments later, we were bundled up and traipsing arm in arm, leaving our footprints down the street and across the field. When we arrived at the nursing home, Grandma's room offered us a warm retreat and priceless memory making.

Grandma lived long enough to put her arms around two of my daughters. By the time my oldest was two, Grandma Mary's room was one of her favorite places to visit. The moment I opened the door to the building, her little feet invariably ran ahead of me, down the hall to Grandma's room. By the time I reached the doorway, these steadfast friends were already snuggled up in each other's' arms and conversation had ensued.

By this time, most of Grandma's verbal skills were gone. My daughters were just beginning to develop, so it was a perfect composition. They had a special way of communicating only they understood. It was amazing to watch. Couple this with the fact they both loved teddy bears and suckers, and their mutual adoration was evident. One of my favorite pictures of these moments is of a precious little pigtailed girl sharing a sucker with her treasured great grandma.

We said goodbye to Grandma on a snowy winter day after her decade long battle with Alzheimer's. No longer were those with dementia referred to as senile, but neither were the issues of their disease fully understood. My mom had dedicated ten years of her life as a caregiver to my grandma. She would be much younger than Grandma when Alzheimer's took up residence in her own life. How could we have known, less than ten years later, Mom would begin her battle with the same disease?

"Because I have a name,
remember I will love you forever."

Warnings From Shore

*The moment we recognize
the reality of this inescapable disease.*

I have been blessed with many strong and wonderful women in my life. There is one last amazing aunt I want you to meet. When I was a child, my great, great Aunt Lennie often wrote me encouraging notes. Our friendship grew as we exchanged letters well into my adulthood. It was one of my greatest pleasures to hear her exuberant voice calling out, "There's my pen pal!" at family gatherings.

I was recently discussing with Auntie how much we miss her. "I have saved every letter she ever wrote me," my auntie shared. I am quite certain I have too, but finding them would require an overhaul of my closet. We recalled the discussion we had on a walk long ago along the shore on the coast. As waves lapped up on the shore, we began to discuss what made Aunt Lennie so special.

She was an amazing woman who possessed rare and wonderful qualities, the kind of woman one wanted to stand close to in hopes of soaking up some of her goodness. Auntie and I liked to believe we were her favorites. It was agreed we would write her a little note sharing these sentiments and enclose a bit of sand in the envelope to be whimsical.

We prepared the envelope and I addressed it: "#1 Great, Great Aunt Lennie." I would be reprimanded if I failed to include #1, which ironically only happened once. Imagine my delight when I visited Aunt Lennie months later to find the bits of sand she had harvested from the envelope in a little bottle by her chair. This sentiment remained there for the rest of her life as a reminder of our adoration. She loved us well and genuinely cherished relationships.

I admire Aunt Lennie for so many reasons and, despite her absence, her life continues to inspire us. She is among the broken hearted mothers who has grieved the loss of a child. Despite losing a young daughter to cancer and an even younger grandson in a tragic accident, she was one of the most positive people I have ever known. By the time this precious woman passed, she had been a widow for decades, stood at the grave of all three of her children, and been shot by a stray bullet while driving the streets of her small, quiet town. What I remember most about her was the smile on her face.

When I was a young mother, this talented woman often shared recipes with me. Visits to her home always included a culinary treat. I can still picture the anticipation on her face as I tasted what she had prepared. When I expressed my enjoyment of the dish (which was a given) a prewritten recipe card was retrieved from a drawer in her kitchen. I would be remiss not to mention her potato soup recipe which won first place. The article from the local newspaper would be included here if space permitted.

One day I was preparing a batch of Aunt Lennie's cornbread salad and called her with a question. "Don't you remember," she said, "we discussed this last year and decided the cornbreads should bake separately." I barely remembered if I had fed the baby that morning. She was amazing. I wanted to be just like her when I "grew up" and told her often. Unfortunately, I descended from her husband's side of the family, resulting in Auntie and I inevitably being introduced as "from Sam's side."

Apparently, this prohibited us from gleaning any of her amazing qualities, at least that is what Aunt Lennie led me to believe. One day I asked what her secret was for living such a joyful life. My beautiful aunt told me she got dressed every morning with the expectation of having a wonderful day. Careful to not overextend herself, she limited her activities. When she no longer had the desire to drive, her car was sold. This meant she could not attend church services, so she dressed in her Sunday best, sat in her chair, and watched it on television.

Have I mentioned she was one hundred years young? My precious aunt, the exemplification of all I seek to be: a woman of courage, outstanding achievements, and noble qualities. However, I am unable to will it, buy it, or produce the same results. If some form of dementia is in our future, it will not be through any fault of our own. Many are destined for a different journey, one requiring Aunt Lennie's grace and resolve to travel.

Aunt Lennie passed away the day after Christmas, a few weeks short of her one hundred and first birthday. No longer would I be able to call her for culinary advice. The recipes she had shared with me would be the extent of those I would ever receive. Her encouragement and expertise, as well as the memories we shared, would live on only in my mind.

The following year, my daughters and I began preparations for our Christmas celebration. Menus were made, schedules discussed, baking days eagerly planned. Some things were a given, like Aunt Lennie's potato casserole and Grandma's cream nut cake. Their advice would never again be a phone call away. I could only hope I had gleaned all that would be required to do these recipes justice.

Mom's Christmas rolls were also a long standing tradition. From the year my parents started dating, she made them for family and friends. Never had a Christmas passed without these rolls gracing our breakfast table Christmas morning. My three daughters had now come to expect them as well. Although Mom usually made them on her own, this particular year we made plans for her to spend a couple of afternoons with us preparing the dough, assembling the rolls, and baking them at our house.

They were quite the undertaking and we were sure she would appreciate the help with the labor intense process. Mom arrived and we set out all the ingredients. As we began to prepare the dough, I asked how we would know when the milk was hot enough. I was met with a blank stare. Later one of the girls said, "Gram, the yeast is clumping up!" "What am I doing wrong?" Seemingly disinterested, Mom turned her attention to something outside the window.

Looking back, it is so blatantly apparent something was terribly wrong. This wonderful cook had made these rolls for over fifty years, yet was unable to offer us one shred of insight. At the time, I was somewhat frustrated Mom was not more interested in the success of this treasured tradition. As I write this over a decade later, tears flow down my face as I experience, once again, the realization that this was the beginning of her long and treacherous journey as a victim of Alzheimer's disease.

The rolls were hardly edible that year. As suddenly as Aunt Lennie's absence in my life took with it her culinary advice, my mother's vast experience in the kitchen had faded as well. One by one, every talent and memory she possessed would be muted. We expect these things to disappear when a loved one leaves this world; however, it is heartbreaking for the person who embodies these attributes to be standing before us, absent of knowledge of things so familiar.

The beginning stage of this infliction is an invaluable season which can be spent understanding our loved one's wishes and getting life in order. Unfortunately, by the time we received Mom's diagnosis, it was too late to discuss her wishes for the future. Her disease progressed well past this stage before we were able to get her the help she needed. In retrospect, it is easy to look at these signs and realize she was experiencing all of them during this time.

This is perhaps one of the greatest gifts we can give our loved one-the gift of time. An early diagnosis is essential if we are to achieve this. If it is suspected your loved one may be experiencing problems, keep a log of what, when, and where these behaviors are happening. This will prove to be a useful tool in helping a doctor determine the diagnosis.

The warning signs of Alzheimer's disease can be subtle. However, after making note of concerns and looking at the overall picture, discrepancies become easier to see. Following are common warning signs published by the Alzheimer's Association. These signs, which occur in no particular order, are easy for me to identify now as I look back at my Mom's symptoms:

1. ***Memory loss that disrupts daily life.*** *One of the most common signs of Alzheimer's, especially in the early stages, is forgetting recently learned information. Others include forgetting important dates or events; asking for the*

same information over and over; relying on memory aides or family members for things they used to handle on their own.

Sometimes forgetting names or appointments, then remembering them later, is normal; frequently forgetting important events is not. Mom planned for and celebrated birthdays enthusiastically. When she began to completely forget our birthdays, it was not only heartbreaking, but a sign of a deeper problem. The year she sent Christmas cards out in early October was a monumental clue something was terribly wrong.

2. ***Challenges in planning or solving problems****. Some people may experience changes in their ability to develop and follow a plan or work with numbers. They may have trouble following a familiar recipe or keeping track of monthly bills. They may have difficulty concentrating and take much longer to do things than they did before.*

We all occasionally make errors in balancing the checkbook or omit an ingredient in a recipe, this is normal. Mom's sudden inability to make her traditional Christmas rolls was a sign this disease had taken over. The challenges she faced in the kitchen, as well as when grocery shopping, produced an overall lack of interest.

3. ***Difficulty completing familiar tasks*** *at home, at work or at leisure. People with Alzheimer's often find it hard to complete daily tasks. Sometimes, people may have trouble*

driving to a familiar location, managing a budget at work or remembering the rules of a favorite game.

It is normal to occasionally need help with the settings on a microwave. My family will confirm; my television remote control struggles are real. However, it was a major clue when my dad began to do the grocery shopping, as well as all the cooking and cleaning. This had always been my mom's area of expertise and she suddenly was not participating at all.

4. **_Confusion with time or place._** *People with Alzheimer's can lose track of dates, seasons and the passage of time. They may have trouble understanding something if it is not happening immediately. Sometimes they may forget where they are or how they got there.*

It is typical, especially after a trip or holiday, to be confused about what day of the week it is. One of the most frustrating warning signs for me was when my mom began to get very angry at me for habitually showing up late or on the wrong day. Even when we wrote our plans down, I could not convince her I had arrived as we had planned.

5. **_Trouble understanding visual images and spatial relationships._** *For some people, having vision problems is a sign of Alzheimer's. They may have difficulty reading, judging distance and determining color or contrast. In*

terms of perception, they may pass a mirror and think someone else is in the room. They may not recognize their own reflection.

Vision problems, such as those due to cataracts, are common as we age. Mom backing the car into a closed garage door was not. When she suddenly abruptly stopped driving, coupled with a bowed out garage door and dented back bumper, it was apparent more than an eye exam was needed.

6. ***New problems with words in speaking or writing.***
People with Alzheimer's may have trouble following or joining a conversation. They may stop in the middle of a conversation and have no idea how to continue or they may repeat themselves. They may struggle with vocabulary, have problems finding the right word or call things by the wrong name.

We all struggle at times to find the right word. My mom had one of the most amazing vocabularies I have ever known and was using words like "shenanigans" well into her disease. The most telltale sign for her was the difficulty in following conversations. She would often withdraw, especially in social gatherings where she might be asked questions.

7. ***Misplacing things and losing the ability to retrace steps.*** *A person with Alzheimer's disease may put things in unusual places. They may lose things and be unable to go*

65

back over their steps to find them again. Sometimes, they may accuse others of stealing. This may occur more frequently over time.

Misplacing things from time to time, such as a pair of glasses or the remote control, happens to all of us. Normally we would not suspect someone of stealing these items. As the disease progressed, my mom became very suspicious and was convinced misplaced items had been stolen.

8. _Decreased or poor judgment._ *People with Alzheimer's may experience changes in judgement or decision making. For example, they may use poor judgment when dealing with money, giving large amounts to telemarketers. They may pay less attention to grooming or keeping themselves clean.*

We have all made a bad decision which we later regret, or ran to the grocery store looking less than impressive. However, when someone like my mom, who was a wonderful seamstress, started choosing shocking combinations of clothing for formal affairs, my suspicions were warranted.

9._Withdrawal from work or social activities._ *A person with Alzheimer's may start to remove themselves from hobbies, social activities, work projects or sports. They may have trouble keeping up with a favorite sports team or remembering how to complete a favorite hobby. They may also avoid being social because of the changes they have experienced.*

Most have us have experienced being weary of work, family and social obligations. I remember early on being frustrated with my normally social mom who seemed to be hiding out in the corner at family gatherings. What I perceived as rude was, in reality, a symptom of my mom's very real struggle with this disease.

10. ***Changes in mood and personality.*** *The mood and personalities of people with Alzheimer's can change. They can become confused, suspicious, depressed, fearful or anxious. They may be easily upset at home, at work, with friends or in places where they are out of their comfort zone.*

Many of us have a very specific way of doing certain things and sometimes become irritable when a routine is disrupted. However, when Mom became convinced her doctor was "playing tricks" on her by telling her his office was located on the fifth floor of a three story building, it became obvious her suspicions were fueled by a more serious problem.

Of course, this disease is full of variables and each person reacts to circumstances differently. However, these warning signs do serve as a good basis for determining if further evaluation should be pursued. It is important to remember a person with this disease did nothing to get it and there is nothing they can do to get out of it.

It is not uncommon to consciously or unconsciously blame the patient. We must remember this disease was not caused by something our loved ones did wrong. They cannot change what is happening and they cannot train it away. Alzheimer's disease is just that, a disease, which is damaging and deteriorating the brain. Research does not support the notion that this disease is caused by a lack of stimulating activities for the brain, nor by eating the wrong foods.

Throughout the years, it has been suggested Alzheimer's disease is caused by everything from inactivity to mental illness. As the Alzheimer's Association likes to say, "It is not possible to do enough crossword puzzles or eat enough kale to reverse the inevitable effects of this deadly disease." This is a disease of the brain. The day will come when causes are uncovered which offer valuable insight into this disease. More research is needed and funding is essential.

Alzheimer's disease is a global problem with staggering, long term costs, but receives only a fraction of the funds other terminal conditions do. It will take billions of dollars in federal funding to fight this disease. The same funding conditions, such as cancer and heart disease research, currently receive. Research has been key in understanding and treating these diseases, and will be necessary in advances in Alzheimer's research as well. This will require the involvement of all of us, as advocates dedicated to finding answers.

"Because I have a name,
please know I did not choose this disease, it chose me."

Waters of Despair

Finding strength, despite adversity,
as circumstances test our resolve.

Regardless of the details of our journey thus far, we have all now converged on this road together. It is critical we learn everything we can about the disease to get the correct diagnosis and medication for our loved ones. This is a gradual process which systematically deteriorates the brain, affecting memory, thinking, and judgement. It is a cruel and lengthy disease and we must be prepared for a long and grueling battle.

There is little hopeful news in this prognosis. Eventually, the brain will no longer be capable of sending appropriate signals to the organs. To date, this disease is incurable and terminal. This is perhaps the most misunderstood aspect of Alzheimer's disease. When my mother died, many people were surprised and would say, "I knew she had Alzheimer's, but I didn't realize she was sick."

This disease must be faced head-on. The first step is to find a doctor with an understanding of the disease process, one experienced in diagnosing dementia diseases, such as Alzheimer's. A capable doctor will guide us through the many options. This journey is not a sprint. We must be ready for many years of navigating the decisions this process presents us.

The gruesome truth is this is a slow, heartbreaking death, stealing memories and function along the way. The good news is it does not have to steal our joy. Until a patient's final breath, there remains a living, breathing human being inside. Despite the forgotten memories, the essence of who the person is remains within, just waiting to be rediscovered. The most important ingredient crucial to our loved one's well-being is our dependable, harmonious, genuine, loving care.

This was the kind of love my dad offered my mom. It was a love that defended his beloved, hid her inadequacies, and took on responsibilities not his own. It was a commitment that believed only the best and was determined to maintain a sense of normalcy in a life of confusion. The weapon which inhibited his plan from being victorious was denial. We all experience it to some extent, but it is imperative it be overcome quickly. Our loved one's well-being is dependent on it and time is of the essence.

After years of hiding my mom's deficiencies, the refusal to accept the realities of this disease was taking its toll on my dad. In his final attempt to escape this horrible truth, Dad took my mom and fled in the middle of the night. I arrived at their home the next morning for an expected visit to find an open suitcase, strewn with clothes, hastily left behind. Suspecting they were headed for their winter retreat on the ocean, I called the landlord there.

After four frantic days, I finally received word they had arrived, although it was obvious they had gotten lost along the way. This would prove to be a tumultuous trip, filled with confusion. Many people urged me to drive down and retrieve my parents. I knew in my heart this was a decision my father needed to make peace with in his own time. Short of tying him up and dragging him out, he would not be willing to make the crucial next steps except by his own accord.

This being said, I do believe there are times decisions must be made for our loved ones, against their wishes. However, in this case, I believed my father deserved my honor and respect for the decisions he was making on behalf of my mom, regardless of how misguided they seemed to me. Ultimately, the experience finally brought my precious dad to the realization Mom needed more support than he alone could provide. He came home, asked me for help, and we were able to get Mom the diagnostic treatment she so desperately needed.

A diagnosis is the first step in getting our loved ones the help they need. Local Alzheimer's Association chapters will have recommendations for doctors experienced in the field of dementia. A neurologist is usually the first stop, and subsequent consultations with a geriatrician or psychiatrist are sometimes necessary. Once a diagnosis is made and medications are prescribed, an experienced internist can usually oversee the patient's care.

It is important to keep a log of specific symptoms to take with you when visiting any doctor. Remember to include when, how often, and where they have occurred. Note any current or previous health problems and bring all medications, including prescriptions, over the counter, and herbal. A physician is only able to treat the symptoms of which they are aware. The more accurate information we can provide, the easier it will be for the doctor to make a diagnosis.

An assessment will then be made, which will be comprised of the patient's medical history and mental status. A series of evaluations measuring memory, reasoning, visual and motor skills, as well as language should be conducted. This will be accompanied by a physical examination and psychiatric evaluation. The family should also be interviewed and asked to provide their insight.

A CAT scan or PET scan is usually the next step. These tests take pictures of the brain and determine if there are changes in the brain indicative of the disease. A PET scan is more comprehensive, measuring brain activity, as well as indicating what parts of the brain are functioning normally. These tests provide useful information that can rule out any other causes, medical or emotional, which might be causing the symptoms.

Early detection is a wonderful gift of time. It affords our loved ones the chance to make their wishes known and participate in planning for the future. Support systems can be put in place, history documented, stories written. Perhaps the most important focus during this time is in making legal and financial decisions. Advance directives, long term healthcare plans, as well as wills should all be created if they haven't been already.

This is a critical time affording those diagnosed with the ability to participate in their own reality for the future. Our loved ones can participate in choosing a team who can provide support and care for them. They can let their wishes be known while they are still able to articulate them. Much positive planning can occur before too many functions are stolen. However, it will not be easy and will require facing reality head-on.

Although certain medications may stall the disease, there is no cure to date. It is my sincerest prayer that readers ten years from now will find my book terribly lacking. "Why was there no mention of the magic pill or the special treatment that cures this disease?" "My loved one has been in remission for five years and their memory is restored." Someday a cure will be found and my book will simply be a historical account of a terrible, obsolete plague that struck millions of Americans.

These writings will one day be a distant reminder of a very bleak account of the past. Perhaps it will be assigned in schools to grasp a better understanding of what this terrible disease was like. The children of the future, having never known a single person inflicted with such a strange and frightening disease. A story so bizarre and unbelievable, they will make fictional movies about this unusual phenomenon. One day. Nothing would thrill me more.

Over ten years ago, my parents and I found ourselves sitting in a neurologist's office numbly staring at a scan projected on the wall. I had been concerned about my mom's health for a few years. She was increasingly forgetful, and even more disturbing, the sweet, cheerful woman I once knew was hardly discernible. She had become suspicious and was often angry over things she perceived, which in reality had not occurred.

Suddenly, phone calls were being answered by my dad. After visiting with me for a few minutes, he would often politely inform me Mom was too busy to talk. I have since come to realize these were exceptionally bad days, riddled with the confusion Dad so desperately did not want me to see. His beloved had to be okay, if only in his mind.

I brought up my concern many times and Dad would quickly discount it. "She is fine! We are all getting older, Judy, and simply don't remember as well as we used to." He did a good job of hiding the severity of her problems and even devised elaborate schemes to keep me from doctor visits. More than once I arrived to accompany them to an appointment only to be told they had gone the day before.

Although I did not want to believe something was wrong, eventually the realities could not be denied. Finally, I called Mom's doctor in desperation but since Mom had not listed me on the permission form, the doctor could not discuss her condition with me. She advised me to accompany my parents to an appointment. My presence in the examination room would be Mom's unspoken acceptance.

However, this particular doctor visit was not about my mom. I had, indeed, forced my presence into this appointment, but she was not the patient on this occasion. My parents and I were emerging from six of the most grueling, traumatic months of our lives. We were fresh from the battlefields, exhausted and heartbroken. My determination to find answers landed us here, receiving a report we neither expected nor wished to receive.

My insistence of stepping into this arena and dispelling my parents' denial had brought us to this fateful day. In just a few short months, this crisis had ultimately handed my mom a diagnosis, forced my parents from their home, and deposited us here, in the office of a neurologist, sitting on a bench, waiting to discuss a PET scan.

Soon we would be called back to the room where a scan of my father's brain would deliver the heartbreaking news.

The doctor sat down with my parents and me to frankly discuss Dad's prognosis and his brain's deterioration. The three of us stared blankly at the scan, attempting to process what was occurring. Finally, the physician said, "I am going to give you a moment to process and will be back to answer any questions you might have." When he left the room, we sat in silence for what seemed like an eternity. I wondered how much more heartache our hearts could bear.

Finally, Mom looked at Dad. He lifted his gaze and looked directly into her eyes, as if searching for a way out of his misery. With deepest concern she said, "Wouldn't it be just awful if that happened to someone?" Terror filled my father's eyes. "It *is* happening to someone! It's happening to *me!*" Those words resonated in me, and over a decade later, still manage to form a lump in my throat.

The day our loved ones were diagnosed is etched in our minds forever. Over a decade after the word dementia was spoken over my father, I can clearly picture the terrified look on my dad's face when he realized something was terribly wrong. There was a part of me which felt guilty for pursuing this. If only we could have just stayed in our blissful state of denial.

It is a day no one wants to experience, but it is an absolute necessity in the process of getting the answers and help our loved one's need. Denial only serves to prolong the inevitable and ultimately makes the process more difficult. Although we did not sign up for this journey, we are on the train and it is headed for an inescapable destination. We can choose to ignore it, deny it, or wish it away but it is our new reality, and will remain so for the duration of our loved one's life.

If there is anything here to be grateful for, I have taken great comfort in knowing my parents' memory of that fateful day, as well as the reality of the news, eventually blissfully disappeared. Ironically, they were laughing and discussing their plans for dinner by the time we had reached the car. It is only on the other side of the diagnosis the process of learning how to facilitate a meaningful life for our loved one throughout the journey can begin.

The doctors and I noticed Dad's confusion while we were seeking answers for my mom. He often got lost while going to her appointments and had a great misperception of time. I told him, "I am here for you, and together we will get Mom the help she needs, but you have to take good care of yourself and stay healthy because I don't know how I could get through this without you!" If only we could command the absence of dementia into existence.

Months before Dad's appointment, as we had suspected, Mom was diagnosed with Alzheimer's disease. The doctors denied her dismissal from the hospital until I secured other living arrangements for my parents. After over forty years in their home, my dad's independence had now been threatened. It would not be without yet another battle. The woman he had been married to for over fifty years was slipping away. His grip was understandably tight on the home they had built together.

Perhaps even more compelling was his desire to not upset or disappoint her. When Dad asked me for help, I promised to be right beside him. His telling response was, "No, could you please handle this? I don't want her to be mad at me." From the time we are very small, we seek to please our parents. Especially as they grow older, we want nothing more than for them to be comfortable, happy, and stress-free. Moving our parents from their place of comfort is hardly the means to achieve this.

However, when dementia darkens the door, safety becomes the utmost concern. Decisions must be made and directions of the doctor must be followed, even at the expense of being perceived as the source of the problem by our loved ones. The beauty of the disease is it is full of grace. Dementia patients are the most forgiving folks you will ever meet.

If we do something today which is not effective, upsets our loved one, even gets us thrown out the door (Unfortunately, I speak from experience here), tomorrow is a new day and we get an instant do-over. As the disease progresses, the next moment often affords us the same benefits. Grudges do not have a long shelf-life in the world of dementia patients.

Not many days passed before I received the call I had been praying for; Dad's voice on the other end saying, "I am not going to fight you on this anymore. Wherever you think we need to go, whatever you think we need to do, we will do it." I had prepared a list of possibilities and was in their driveway before Dad had a chance to change his mind. By that afternoon we had toured some beautiful facilities and signed a contract for their new home.

Now, suddenly, I was spending every day with my parents through the process of closing down their home. Over the course of the next few weeks I overheard Dad's investment conversations on the phone. He would state he was confused, could not find the paperwork, and was unable to make a decision. A few moments later I could hear him reciting his credit card number.

This was happening on a daily basis, so I began answering their phone when I could. Unfortunately, I discovered many other things threatening my parents' financial independence. As I continued to seek the advice of Mom's doctors to get her stabilized and on the right medications, I researched and worked behind the scenes to determine what was happening in Dad's world.

The severity of my father's problems was discovered when it became apparent he was a victim of a terrible scam. What I discovered had the potential to financially devastate my parents. Ultimately, I had no choice but to follow through with plans Dad had made years before, actions I promised to carry out in events such as these. Boldly, yet reluctantly, I filed for power of attorney for both my parents, taking on all of their personal and financial decisions.

This was a heart-wrenching season of life when I realized the wise, witty man I turned to for advice and called on for reassurance was gone. Lost, as well, was the loving mom who supported me through every triumph, disappointment, and important moment in my life. The couple standing before me, which bore a striking resemblance to my parents, could no longer fill those shoes. I was making the most critical decisions I had ever made and the two people I had leaned on and counted on the entirety of my life had vanished, seemingly overnight.

As I grieved the parents I once knew, I was left to begin the process of learning to forge a relationship anew with these familiar looking individuals whose actions and thoughts were not familiar to me and who reacted to me in unpredictable ways. I needed help. This road could not be navigated on my own. I phoned the Alzheimer's Association in desperation, searching for answers. My lifeline on the other end of the phone was a comforting voice who has now been a dear friend for over a decade.

She came to my home and spent over three hours with me, arming me with the strength and understanding I would need to take the next steps. I have sought her insight and support many times since to guide me through critical decisions which had to be made over the past decade. This dear friend is the founder of Caregiver Connection, which provides counseling and care consultation to help families make informed decisions for their loved one's care.

The most important step we can take for ourselves at this point is to connect with someone experienced in the field of dementia who can guide us through these decisions. Finding a local support group where information can be shared and connections made with others who are on this journey is also invaluable. Especially in the beginning stages of this disease, the details and decisions can be overwhelming. We have been presented with a crisis, which must be dealt with at the same time we are grieving a relationship which has now changed.

Although exhaustion is common and time becomes a precious commodity, it is important to make a commitment early on to take care of yourself. Caregivers are at an increased risk of health issues due to the stress and demands this disease places on them. Your loved one will only benefit from your care if you remain healthy enough to do so. You are not alone. Many are on this journey and you will benefit from sharing ideas, concerns, and information.

The Alzheimer's Association provides classes and seminars which provide valuable information, as well as the opportunity to connect with other family members. They will also be able to connect you with local support groups. The time spent is a wise investment beneficial to you, as well as your loved one. Some of my strongest support and dearest friendships have been born in these groups. The camaraderie we share is undeniable.

When you are the primary caregiver for someone with dementia, this will present the unique challenge of finding care for them while you are away. Allow others to help: family members, friends, and other trusted assistance. You will find people want to help, yet often do not know how. Make a list of needs and be ready to let them be known when you are offered assistance.

There are also many options for respite in local adult day care centers. The Alzheimer's Association relayed a story of a daughter who came up with a brilliant idea when her father was reluctant to participate in the program. Because this man always provided for his family, it was upsetting when he could no longer contribute. After moving into his daughter's household, she cleverly arranged with the care facility for her father to obtain a job.

A clever routine ensued. She dropped her dad off in the morning, slipping an envelope of cash to an employee. Her father was assigned little chores throughout the day. At the end of the week, he received his pay, an envelope of cash, which he gave to his daughter, saying, "Go buy some groceries with this." She put it back in her purse, ready to continue this cycle the following week.

Find opportunities to continue doing things you enjoy. A friend once described her weekly afternoon away from her husband, who had been diagnosed with Alzheimer's, as an opportunity to gather sunshine. She said after taking time for herself to do something enjoyable, this enabled her to return refreshed. We will become irritable and fatigued if we do not learn to recharge ourselves. Make a commitment to gather sunshine on a regular basis to nurture yourself, and in turn, light your loved one's world.

*"Because I have a name,
don't feel guilty when you can't provide everything I need.*

Rocky Shores

Helping our loved ones to a place of safety
by placing their well-being above their will.

One beautiful spring morning many years ago, I was
driving down a familiar city street. Traffic was
congested and moving quickly, challenging the forty-five
mile per hour speed limit. Daydreaming about the
responsibilities I was accomplishing, my car continued
traveling in the left lane by the median. Suddenly, a car
turned, coming straight towards me. I desperately looked
to my right and found no opportunity to change lanes.

As the car approached, I could see the driver was a grey
haired man. What affected me most was he apparently
had no idea he was traveling towards oncoming traffic.
Horns attempted to alert him of his mistake as he
continued his pursuit. For a moment, time seemed to be
frozen as I experienced the realization he could crash into
me head-on and kill me. In a split second, thankfully, cars
next to me quickly reacted and slowed down, which
allowed me into the other lane.

The elderly man continued up the road, seemingly
completely unaware he was driving down the wrong side
of the street. As I later reflected on this horrifying
moment, it was equally as frightening to realize my father,

still driving city streets, could potentially kill someone. I was horrified to think of him being jailed for injuring someone, or killed himself, because I had not yet intervened.

Tragedy was averted that day, but the severity of my personal situation remained. My daughters had become fearful of riding with Pop and reported he drove extremely fast. I became concerned and devised a plan to witness his driving skills for myself. I called him one morning to ask if he could give me a ride while my car was getting an oil change. He willingly picked me up and agreed to take me to a few stops along the way. Surprisingly, he drove at a snail's pace, well below the speed limit, the entire way.

Other family members and I followed Dad on occasion after learning he was frequently getting lost. I found no evidence of incompetence until one particular day while filling a prescription for my mom. The pharmacist recognized me and said she needed to tell me about my dad's recent visit. She started to speak, and then openly wept as she relayed the account of my father, shaking and scared, asking to use the phone.

She told me he had lost his car in the parking garage. After searching for over an hour, he finally found his way to the pharmacy on foot. She said Dad called my mom and said, "Please don't worry. I am okay and will find my car and be home soon." It was at that moment I realized my father was now shielding me from the reality of his own disease. My eyes stared into the pharmacist's tear soaked eyes, pleading to be rescued as well.

Coming to the realization a loved one no longer has the capacity to drive is one challenge. Implementing a change, by taking their car keys, is another matter altogether. One of Dad's doctors adamantly told me he absolutely should not be driving, another was reluctant to get involved and said it was not my decision to make. Ultimately, regardless of the opinions of others, it is our responsibility to get those with dementia to the safety of shore.

It is amazing to me that most states automatically renew driver's licenses without testing. Meaning decades after the young teenager successfully completes a driving exam, they can still be behind the wheel of a car as a senior citizen without any further training. Some states require an eye exam, even fewer implement the requirement of a written test at a certain age. Illinois is currently the only state to mandate that drivers retake a road test as they age. The responsibility will likely rest on you to take the steps necessary when it is no longer safe for your loved one to drive.

There are resources available which can evaluate a senior's driving skills. Doctors can administer a CDR, or Clinical Dementia Rating, scale which measures driving competence. They are also able to order a road test through The Department of Transportation. Additionally, AAA has an interactive driving evaluation, which is conducted at home. When possible, it is best to let the decision come from a state department or doctor so you will not be perceived as the enemy.

Seniors age eighty and older have the highest rate of fatal crashes per year. Couple this statistic with the loss of cognitive function dementia mandates and the recipe for tragedy is obvious. Silver Alerts are frequent and pose yet another reason for concern. Most drivers with dementia get lost on routine, caregiver-sanctioned trips to usual locations. Sadly, most are found in a different county or state. The absence of sound reasoning skills will usually inhibit those suffering with dementia from recognizing their inability to safely drive.

Cars represent freedom and independence, so the topic will have to be approached delicately and creatively. My dad's history in his family owned auto dealership imposed deep convictions when it came to the subject of his car. Dad was the only person in his high school class to have a car, far be it for me to take one away now. He did not intend to part with his, nor the independence it afforded him. Ultimately, my concern for his safety soon outweighed my fear of disappointing or upsetting my dad.

I recalled my granddad removing the battery from his sister's car years before when it became apparent she could no longer safely drive. His plan worked beautifully. She could see her car in the driveway and even relayed stories of driving around town long after the car was no longer operable. From my previous experience of being tossed out the door, I knew a confrontation with Dad would not be effective. My granddad was a clever man, so I determined to implement this idea.

By this point, dad had lost his car keys several times and even occasionally forgot how to start the car. In these instances, he called the local dealership and had his car towed, thinking it was in need of a repair. My hope was he would soon tow the car again when it no longer started because of a loosened wire. I would then quietly sell his

91

beloved car. I talked to the dealership and they agreed to simply tell Dad a part was being ordered if he called to inquire. These are the desperate decisions I made in those harrowing days.

Unfortunately, for whatever reason, Dad did not have his car towed. Therefore, it sat disabled for some time, as a source of great frustration and anguish. Eventually Uncle Bill persuaded me to sell Dad's treasured possession. With great anguish, I reconnected the wire and drove his car away feeling deceitful. I was riddled with guilt and felt as if I was the most terrible daughter in the world. This was confirmed the next day when I arrived at my parents' retirement home to find a police officer taking a report on Dad's stolen car.

As terrible as this decision was and as calloused as it sounds, my motivation was concern for my parents' safety. I allowed Dad to go through the misery of not understanding why his car would not run any longer in exchange for a greater cause: The certainty he would not have to go through the terror of getting horribly lost, hurt, or endangering someone else. My father had lost the reasoning skills required to understand the wisdom in the decision which had to be made.

I have come to realize it is sometimes better when things just slip away. Even when an agreement is made, too often it is curiously gone the next moment and all deals are off. The skills required for driving will quickly diminish with the challenges of dementia; the reasoning skills required are too numerous. Sadly, it is not a question of if your loved one can safely drive, rather it is a matter of when their safety will be placed above their will.

This was definitely one of the most heart-wrenching decisions I made. I take great comfort in knowing that in doing so I kept Dad, as well as those around him, safe. Driving is a huge safety concern, yet even without a car the world is full of hazards for those with dementia to navigate. There are plenty of dangers in a home and even more outside its four familiar walls.

As I discovered several years ago, one's own two feet can be equally as dangerous as their presence behind the wheel of a car. While driving home one lovely spring day, I noticed a well-dressed, beautiful woman. Despite her slight frame, confidence and determination exuded from her. Every well-placed step she took was sure. Even so, it was apparent the walker she pushed was a necessary aide.

Over her arm she carried a purse, much too large for her frame. Its contents, one could easily assume, were the usual assortment of lipsticks, a billfold with cash for her outing, and other personal necessities. It was obvious she was on a very important mission and I would not have bothered her at all, had she not been walking down the middle of this very busy city street.

Before I even noticed this dear woman, the swerving cars in the distance caught my attention. Must be a dead animal or large piece of debris in the road, I assumed. As I drew closer, the sound of horns and screeching tires brought a sense of urgency to the otherwise calm day. Horror raced through me when I saw this white haired woman making her way up the road, oblivious to the traffic around her. My friend-to-be remained insouciant and untroubled, seemingly unaware of the imminent danger surrounding her.

I am not sure I would advise what I did next, but even in retrospect I cannot think of a more favorable alternative. Flipping on my hazards, I stopped just short of the skid marks a swerving car ahead of me had left in its wake. Traffic continued unconcerned, albeit a bit irritated, I'm sure, at my inconvenient and discourteous parking spot. As I opened my door, I remember briefly considering the

94

dangerous position in which I was placing myself. These considerations, however, were fleeting. This woman was in extreme danger and I was on a mission.

Olivia, the woman I was yet to meet, was my only concern at the moment. I abandoned my car in the middle of the road and approached her. Walking beside her, I greeted her and asked if I could help. Thankfully, she was receptive to my offer and did not seem the least bit suspicious or frightened. Although she had no idea of the dangerous position we were in, she confided she was growing a bit tired from her walk and would be thankful for a ride. We turned and walked back toward my car, with quite the audience of passing cars. I helped this slight woman into the front seat and, once she was safely inside, put her walker in the back.

Although relieved for my newest friend to be out of harm's way, I did not have the slightest idea what to do with her next. If I am completely honest, I have to admit I was a bit concerned a passerby might by phoning in a report of an abduction. I drove to a nearby neighborhood and turned off the busy road, parking safely by the side of the road. The more quickly I could ascertain where she lived, the sooner she would be home. I was quite sure someone was missing this dear lady.

"I'm Judy," I said. "Lovely to meet you," she said, "my name is Olivia." Although there were certainly issues which caused this dear woman to put herself in harm's way, she seemed alert. I assumed she would be able to tell me where she lived. Unfortunately, this was not the case and it quickly became apparent Olivia had dementia. I knew the neighborhood well and could think of no senior facility in the area. At this point, I called the police, in hopes someone had reported her missing.

While we were waiting for the police to arrive, Olivia told me she was headed for the ice cream shop. I was familiar with the store, which was about two miles in the opposite direction. I asked if her address or any clues to help me get her home might be in her purse. She was eager to show me its contents. As I had suspected, her purse was well stocked, but not as I had imagined. She opened the large black bag to reveal dozens of business cards. They appeared to be from every doctor, medical facility, and business office she had visited in the last several years.

Since Olivia's purse offered no clues as to her identity or address, when the police officer arrived, we began the process of calling phone numbers on the business cards. The cards were portioned out as the officer and I began the process of these tricky conversations. "Hello, I have found a woman and am hoping you might know her. Have you ever shined Olivia's teeth?" Our sweet fugitive remained unflustered and seemed somewhat entertained by our antics.

There are a variety of reasons those with dementia leave the comforts of their home. They almost never realize they are placing themselves in harm's way. Even with cars darting around her, Olivia seemed unaware. Couple the challenges of dementia with loss of hearing, an unsteady gait, or vision problems, and this lack of supervision becomes a very serious problem.

The officer finally found a doctor's office which identified an elderly patient named Olivia who matched our fugitive's description. Thankfully, the receptionist was willing to give us the number of a niece living out of state. When we reached her by phone, it was discovered Olivia did live in a memory care center, almost a mile away. It is still incomprehensible to me this senior had made it that far without coming across anyone concerned enough to help.

Equally as alarming was the reaction of the staff upon Olivia's return. Although obviously glad to see her and relieved to have her home, they had absolutely no idea she was missing. Olivia had been with me at least forty-five minutes and I suspect it took her at least that long to have walked as far as she had navigated. I made certain staff knew Olivia would like some ice cream as I hugged her goodbye. She smiled sweetly and eagerly followed her caregiver to enjoy the treat she had most definitely earned.

The officer urged the facility to get a security bracelet for Olivia immediately. Monitoring devices are readily available for the elderly; many now incorporate GPS. At the very least, facilities should have alarms in place which signal when a person with a security bracelet has passed through an exterior door. In a home setting where an alarm system is not practical, an ID bracelet is imperative. Any safeguard ensuring the safe return of your loved one is more important than you will ever know until they are missing.

"Because I have a name, please keep me safe
when I no longer can navigate decisions on my own."

Sifting Through Sand

Making necessary living decisions and
choosing treasured possessions for the journey.

Early in the disease process it will no longer be safe for
your loved one to be left alone. Whether this comes at
the demand of a doctor or due to a series of dangerous
mishaps, the decision to make a change is never easy.
We must sift through the options and gather the
components which will provide the best quality of life for
our loved ones. Those with dementia believe they can
take care of themselves. Even if one stays in their home
and caregivers are brought in, expect any adjustment to
be met with great resistance.

If it is determined your loved one can manage at home for
the time being, it is imperative to reassess safety in all
rooms. Accidents must be anticipated and avoided
before they occur, not unlike preparing a home for a little
one's visit. As much as we want to believe in our loved
one and trust they are capable, this disease
unfortunately will continue to steal the reasoning
necessary to live independently.

Memory problems invite a host of safety issues, such as
forgotten candles, meals left in the oven, or unattended
bathtub filling with water. Although the understanding

of how to turn the stove on to heat water for tea may still be intact, this task has a variety of safety concerns. Disconnecting the stove so it cannot be used is one option. This will dictate an even higher level of overseeing and facilitating meals.

As I experienced, driving is also a serious concern. It is not simply a matter of if our loved one can remember who they are and where they live that dictates whether they are capable of driving themselves to the store and back. Driving requires an understanding of traffic laws, signs, emergency conditions, as well as perception of time and distance. Those with dementia will very quickly lose the ability to safely drive.

Perhaps one of the greatest concerns is medication. Dementia patients quite often are on a combination of several powerful prescriptions, along with medications they may be taking for other conditions. Due to the challenges those with dementia face, the dependable administration of medication will require outside assistance and monitoring. Many factors will need to be considered when deciding on living arrangements, including financial considerations, proximity to family members, and other health issues.

It is important to stay a step ahead of this disease and anticipate future decisions. A person with dementia who lives alone will need frequent assessments and daily visits. Expect their needs to change, with more care becoming necessary. Common needs to anticipate in the early stages of the disease are: reminders to eat and assistance in preparing meals; as well as help with grooming, running errands, and daily chores. A plausible option early in the disease may be to bring full or part time help into the home.

Although this will afford the individual less upheaval, as well as familiar surroundings, do not expect the transition to be without its own set of challenges. Finding someone your loved one will accept is key. Several caregivers may need to be interviewed and vetted out before a plausible choice is found. Ask for referrals and speak with these families to gain recommendation and information about the applicant. It is important to note, individuals completing Home Health Aide training have taken specialized classes and must meet certain requirements to keep their certification.

There are many agencies which provide care, as well as private caregivers who can be found through referrals in your local support group. Bringing a stranger into your loved one's home is not an easy proposition and will require a great deal of overseeing from you. This being said, I would be remiss if I failed to mention this was my primary option of care for many years.

When I moved my parents from their home, the severity of my father's problems was still unknown. Therefore, the retirement community we chose was an independent living facility. Very quickly it was apparent more supervision and assistance would be necessary. Moving my parents again, after a contract was signed, was impractical. Not to mention, I am not certain any of us would have survived another upheaval at that point.

After a series of caregivers sent from local agencies was unsuccessful, I asked for referrals at the retirement facility. The first person I called did not have room in her schedule to help us, but because I was going out of town, agreed to come over the weekend. When she met my Dad, he reminded her of her own father. Miraculously, after tossing more than a few caregivers out the door and refusing others entrance into the apartment, Dad took a liking to her as well. His acceptance was a remarkable surprise.

She agreed to stay and faithfully provided loving care for many years. As Mom's health and mental facilities declined, more help was necessary. Other caregivers were recommended and soon we had a team of four beautiful women providing my parents the assistance they needed. A beautiful woman named Tammy completed this group of dedicated professionals. Ultimately, she walked for over a decade with us as an advocate for my parents, and support for me as I maneuvered the often treacherous shores of this journey.

This option is not inexpensive, but with two parents requiring care, it was a plausible alternative to the cost of memory care. It proved to be a credible option for us for many years. The ladies caring for my parents became like family to us, participating in our holidays, family dinners, birthday parties, and weddings. As an only child with this immense responsibility, their commitment was invaluable to me. Every situation is different and the decision will be intensely personal.

Regardless of what is chosen, you will need the support of others. The greatest need for this support will be when caring for a loved one in your home. Support from other family members, as well as their understanding of your loved one's needs will be crucial. This option will likely mean a significant change in your daily life and will require a great deal of patience, resolve, and understanding. Due to the challenges and expense of outside care, many families choose to care for their loved one themselves. This is a wonderful, selfless option with many benefits.

The most obvious blessing is the gift of time this affords you with your loved one. One of my dear friends has moved her mother-in-law, JoAnn, into their home. She educates herself about her medical needs and provides the care that is needed. The stories she shares about their relationship, which was close before and even more special now, warm my heart. Although challenging issues will be inevitable, a value cannot be placed on these priceless moments.

Because of the immensity of this responsibility, some family members share in the care. This often means their loved one must move from home to home periodically. This offers fresh energy and reprieve, but also dictates a constant state of transition. Coupled with the issues dementia presents, it is often a challenge to provide security and consistency. Ultimately, one family may be better suited to take on the responsibility while other family members provide respite for the primary caregiver, as well as financial support. Outside assistance will likely be necessary when caring for a loved one long-term.

It is a difficult proposition, but changes in living arrangements will have to be made. Whatever the decision, do not expect change to be without challenge. Although our loved ones may realize things are going awry, most will likely not recognize it as the result of their own inadequacies. Problems may often be perceived to be as the result of someone, or something, else. Ultimately, we will be the guide in helping our loved ones adjust and decide which precious treasures will accompany them on the journey.

The progression of the disease, medical issues, and hospital stays all threaten a change in feasible living options. Additionally, because of Medicare rules and regulations, options may decrease as the patient's medical issues persist. It is important to note certain criteria must be met to gain acceptance in a memory care facility. Once a patient is unable to bear weight, they are referred to other facility types. One fall could instantly change the options available.

Thankfully, individuals are not currently forced to move out of a facility due to physical conditions. This is referred to as the right to "age in place." Because of this law, once an individual makes their home in a memory care facility, a fall or failing health would not force a move to another facility type. It should also be noted facilities, as well as state agencies, have different rules and regulations regarding outside care which will need to be explored before making any decision.

Although there are many facilities equipped to care for the elderly, dementia patient care requirements are unique. For this reason, memory care facilities provide the most comprehensive care for your loved one. Overall, they have a better understanding of the care those with memory impairments require. Look for one with a smaller, or separate communities. Those with dementia are easily overwhelmed in large groups and spaces.

Many facilities are now built to resemble a home with a commons area and kitchen in a central location. Fewer halls offer less of an opportunity to get lost or overwhelmed. Additionally, memory care facilities should be secure and conducive for dementia patients. Look for calming spaces, low patient to aide ratios, and activity programs based on research specific to the diseases of dementia. An added benefit to this type of facility is the friendship and support you will find in the kindred spirits of other family members. The essence of any home is composed of those who live within. Those with dementia usually find comfort in small groups of other folks with similar abilities.

A memory care facility is just one participant in the team comprising your loved one's care. You are an invaluable, integral part of any living option's success. Your loved one needs you, as an advocate, a source of information, and a transporter of sunshine from beyond the walls. Communicate with those providing your loved one's care. Let them know what your loved one's likes and interests are. The more they know about the unique individual they are caring for; the better quality of care they can provide.

The vast majority of those working as memory care providers have their patients' best interest at heart. Most are loving, caring individuals who treat those they serve like a family member. However, it takes many team members and a great deal of coordination to provide the care our loved ones will need. No facility is perfect; things will be forgotten and overlooked. The road ahead will require a great deal of commitment, understanding, and grace.

In my quest for the best care possible for my parents, I have not been afraid to ask questions and voice concerns. However, I always sought to do so with respect. We are on the same team and the best possible life for our loved one should be our common goal. We must be a part of the solution. Above all, when issues arise, do not have discussions in front of your loved one. Work to make their life as peaceful and stress-free as possible.

Understanding the changes this disease may present in the future and choosing a living option requiring the least amount of transition is crucial. Moving is not easy, especially for those suffering with dementia. Familiarity is important to their well-being and feelings of security. The more continuity our loved one is afforded, the more positive their experiences will be.

When I began discussing a move with my parents, due to the insistence of Mom's doctor, both flatly refused. They had lived in their home for over forty years and had no intention of leaving. It was especially difficult because I was dealing with not one, but two, determined individuals. After much tribulation, and most likely due to Dad's fatigue from living with Mom's confusion on a daily basis, he finally agreed.

Dad and I spent an afternoon touring apartments, drinking smoothies, and discussing his opinions of resident dogs. I researched beforehand and had narrowed the options down to a few of the most plausible choices. Victory was achieved when my dad chose a new home, without being overwhelmed by too many options. Although this would have been a harrowing experience for Mom, one she would not have enjoyed, it was important for Dad to have some control over the situation.

He weighed the choices, signed the papers, and in the end felt the decision had been his alone. Subsequently, I took a few of the paint color samples to Mom. We had a wonderful time discussing the options and ultimately she chose the wall color for their new apartment. Our loved ones should participate, when they can, in their own destinies. For all the absolutes out of their control, it is essential those whose lives are most affected be allowed to participate.

Although I managed to facilitate some positive experiences during the move, I failed terribly at times. When I began the overwhelming process of packing and moving my parents, my approach often resembled a freight train. For weeks, I arrived each morning to continue rambling through my parents' home with moving boxes and tape. I shudder when I think of the dining room table I used to display items which I planned to dispose of in a garage sale. Understandably, there was an enormous amount of work to be done, and they could not take everything with them.

However, in retrospect, I realize much of this process should not have been carried out in my parents' presence. It only served to confuse and upset them. One day I walked into the kitchen of my parents' home and found them gleefully unloading a box of dishes I had recently packed. They were discussing where the dishes should be stored. "How about putting the plates up here?" my mom asked, opening an empty cabinet. "That would be fine," Dad responded, as he moved dishes from the box onto the shelf.

I stood behind them in horror. Was this really happening? They were well aware they were moving, weren't they? The scene was shockingly reminiscent of my mother's experience during my grandma's move. These struggles are traumatic, at best. For the first time, I was grasping the magnitude of my mother's heartache all those years ago. Depending on the development of the disease and the capabilities they possess, many of our loved ones will be faced with the heartbreaking challenge of processing the reality many times over.

Looking back, it is nothing short of a miracle we survived this tumultuous season. The move was filled with heartache and challenges, which were greatly the product of my incessant attempts to reason with my parents. I was still communicating with them as if they had the capacity to rationalize the situation. Not only were they heartbroken each time they processed the surprise of a move, there was now a bossy "child" sorting through their precious belongings.

On one occasion I was taking inventory of furniture to determine what would fit in their new home. After mapping out a place for Dad's desk, I moved onto Mom's sewing room. Although she no longer could sew, I knew her sewing machine was immensely important to her. After unsuccessfully finding a place on my hand drawn floor plan for it, I mentioned I could keep it at my home. She became inconsolably upset. "This is exclusively mine," she insisted. "I am so sorry, Mom. It was wrong of me to suggest such a thing."
There are so many things I would have done differently during my parent's move if given the opportunity. I was

just beginning to understand the disease process myself. Mom definitely should have been spared from witnessing the upheaval of her home. The countless boxes of treasures would not have been missed had she simply been settled beforehand. Dad was a trickier proposition. He was still driving at the time and continued to return to their house even after the move. As a result, many loads of belongings, having neither place nor function, were transported to their small apartment.

The weeks leading up to the move proved to be challenging. Mom was especially troubled with my interference in their lives and apparent intent on disrupting their home. One morning I arrived to continue the packing process. I turned the corner of my childhood home to walk in my father's office and noticed my portrait was missing. I stopped in my tracks and turned to examine the somewhat yellowed rectangular shape which now inhabited the wall my image had graced since I was four. I asked Dad what had happened to it. He simply responded, "Your mother is very upset with you."

A few days later, I received a call from Dad late one evening. He insisted I come quickly. "It's an emergency!" he said. I raced to their house as possible horrible scenarios dashed through my mind. I knew I should have gotten my parents out of the house sooner. A promise was made to the doctor I would have them moved quickly. This process was monumental and taking longer than I anticipated. Regardless, I should have never left them alone in the house.

My car had barely reached the driveway before I saw my frantic father emerge from the door inside the garage. He was running, more quickly than I had seen in years, towards my car. Why had I not gathered more information over the phone? I was sure an ambulance should have been called. I swung open my door and bolted towards my father. His image emerged from the shadows. What was he carrying?

A bundle, wrapped in a blanket was in his arms. My heart sank, knowing this must be my mother and fearing the worst. As he approached, he heaved the carefully covered bundle into my arms, then sprinted back towards the garage. I braced myself as the blanket was flung with full force into my body. To my surprise, it was much lighter than I imagined. Not light by any means, but definitely not the weight of a human body as I was expecting.

"Put it in your car!" my father yelled from the shadows. "We must work quickly!" As I shoved the mysterious blanket clad package into the back of my car, I lifted the edge to reveal what was so terribly important to my dad. It was his own beloved portrait, painted in the likeness of his much younger image. This treasured representation of a handsome, distinguished man had graced the wall of his home office, possibly since the day we first called this place home.

Tears filled my eyes as I realized how much we had lost; how cruel this thief had been to us. Why did this disease have to strike our family, not only once, but twice? Never had I felt so alone. I was raising my three daughters on my own and wearing the title of only child, thanks to my brother's murder. I turned to see this scared and troubled man frantically running back to me. "I got yours, too," he said. "Take them, save them before she burns them!" I watched as his defeated frame cowered back towards the garage. He turned as he reached the door. "Go! You've got to get out of here!"

Hiding our images was the only way my mom had of expressing the fear and anguish she felt from the changes this disease was forcing us to carry out. Those pictures are a testimony the emotions of those with dementia are intact, regardless of their inability to articulate them. The distinguished painting of my dad was the only tangible evidence he had of his past and he protected it fiercely. For over a decade to come, it proudly graced the wall of his retirement home. Very late in his disease, he was capable of identifying the handsome man in the portrait.

My childhood portrait has hung on private walls of my home since this troubling night. She is tucked beside closet shelves, or hung in my tiny craft room above my mother's sewing machine. Discrete, yet not hidden. Her cherished message is exclusively mine. The child in the photo silently reminds me just how fragile life is. She whispers prayers of hope and promises of unfailing love. The image of the little girl looking back at me, immensely treasured by her parents, reminds me how precious love is.

"Because I have a name, regardless of where I live, please visit me often and never stop loving me."

Building Sandcastles
The tedious and beautiful process
of creating a home in which to thrive.

Most of us are resistant to change of any kind, especially when it comes in the form of an unwelcome transition. A disruption in living arrangements is especially difficult for those with dementia. Diminishing cognitive function, which affects the ability to understand, coupled with loss of control over their fate, is understandably upsetting. By this point in the disease, it is likely a move will soon be experienced, if it has not been already. Although some will acclimate quickly, be prepared for the process of settling into a new home to take up to six months.

Frustration and confusion are common feelings which are often disguised as anger. Unfortunately, family members usually get the brunt of these outbursts. This may be the result of being perceived as one who can fix, or is responsible for, the problem. Perhaps we simply serve as a reminder of past living situations. Whatever the case, ask those providing care how they perceive your loved one to be adapting. You may be surprised to find they are doing quite well when you are not around.

I liken the process of creating a living space to building sandcastles, in that each is a unique representation of its proprietor. I am always amazed when I stop to admire intricate sandcastles found along the beach. These creations are labors of love, usually representing many hours of effort. Often the swimsuit clad architects responsible for these creations can be found nearby. You will recognize them by the look of pride displayed on their faces. This is what your loved one's room represents for them.

Years of developing an identity, interests, a uniqueness not found in any other individual, should be reflected in their surroundings. I am not suggesting cluttering the room with every mug collected through the years or countless trophies and awards accumulated over decades. What I am recommending is this: anyone who enters the room should instantly be able to recognize a rare and wonderful individual. Something meaningful about this unique person should be communicated the moment visitors enter their room.

My Dad loved to travel, which afforded my parents many wonderful memories. On Dad's eightieth birthday, I mounted a collection of photos from their adventures in one sizable frame. Each picture was labeled with a point of reference. This gave guests at his party a topic of conversation; it was also a source of pride for my Dad. This beautiful sentiment was subsequently hung in my parents' apartment. It introduced all who entered to the unique and adventurous couple residing there.

Think about your loved one's interests or hobbies, past or present, and their most precious memories. If he had an interest in cars, enjoyed traveling, or she had the most beautiful flower garden on the block, incorporate this into the decor. Perhaps a beloved pet or favorite animal's image is representative of a special memory. If cooking was their specialty, a beautiful wall mural of a kitchen scene could be included in the room.

Be assured, their most treasured connection is you, regardless of how you are being treated at the moment. For this reason, family photos should be considered. A collage of eight to ten photos in frames of various sizes is one example of an esthetically pleasing display. When hung on the wall, it will be uncluttered and easily viewed. Photographs of meaningful moments will encourage beautiful memories, as well as conversation with guests.

Several years ago I was visiting my parents when a caregiver noticed our family photograph. Smiling back at her were the images of my beautiful parents, as well as a tall, teenage boy. Sitting on my father's lap was a tiny, blonde headed girl with a crooked smile. Because my brother was so much older, it was often suggested that I was not planned. This assumption most usually bore the label of mistake or surprise. Since I was brought home on my brother's ninth birthday, I found surprise to be most complimentary.

These less than sensitive comments seemed to insult my parents. When such a remark was made, they were quick to correct. "Oh, no, we always wanted a little girl," they would say. My glowing disposition had certainly been worth the wait. I found it odd that anyone would question this; obviously my parents were delighted to have me. This blissful interpretation continued for decades, right up to the point when my parents were stripped of all filters.

"What a beautiful picture of your family," the caregiver commented. Dad examined the photograph, then pointed to the precious toddler perched on the lap of his much younger image. "That one right there," he chuckled, "we sure weren't counting on her!" I looked up in horror from my seat beside Mom, as I processed the image of my amused father. Taking a deep breath, I

119

paused before examining my mother's face, in desperate search of a glimmer of hope. She laughed in agreement, "She was a big surprise!"

Dementia not only clouds present realities, it is also capable of successfully uncovering some of the deepest and most hidden secrets ever kept. Eventually, the sudden realization of the facts surrounding my existence became one of my most treasured truths. How grateful I am to have been allowed this life, as well as the opportunity to care for my parents in their most trying years.

The insight I have gained in the process has taught me much about life and love. Regardless of what our loved ones are facing, the essence of who they are, as well as the accumulation of the experiences they have had, still exist. Now dependent on us to help uncover these truths for them, they count on us to display these unique and wonderful qualities. The perspective of who they are, and pride they feel as a result of these views, will largely be understood through the reminders we incorporate in their room.

Before your loved one is brought to their new home, the space should be carefully arranged. Life with dementia is confusing enough; your loved one will not function well with the chaos and clutter of moving boxes. It is impossible to accomplish this on your own. Help will need to be recruited to facilitate a meaningful outing for your loved one while moving is taking place. A familiar chair, regardless of how tattered it may be, or favorite quilt in peaceful, orderly surroundings should be an instant point of recognition when they arrive.

The goal is to reduce as much of the inevitable stress of moving as possible, while preparing a space which feels familiar. This means resisting the temptation to buy new furniture or bedding. It may seem reasonable to assume updated items would be a welcome change. However, in this situation, familiar equals peace of mind. To achieve this, it is helpful to take pictures of the existing home before anything is moved. Creating a new room which closely resembles the previous living space will provide a priceless feeling of comfort and security.

The room should be filled sparingly with well-loved and recognized items. Although their previous home may have been stuffed to the brim, at this point, less is definitely more. Most items will not be missed in their absence. However, I suggest you wait to dispose of questionable items until several months after the move. I placed everything of possible importance into boxes to be stored in my attic. Months later, when I was clear minded, I sorted through the boxes and made those decisions.

This arrangement has an additional advantage. If by chance something of significance is overlooked, you will be able to orchestrate a magical reappearance. The process will be a monumental undertaking, as you sift through treasures usually representing decades of memories. Grant yourself a little grace. These difficult decisions are being made at a stressful, emotion-filled period in our lives. Everything does not have to be decided this second. Your loved one's well-being is top priority, taking precedence over stuff. I mean treasures, of course.

Items of great value: wedding rings, expensive watches, or anything holding great sentimental value are best kept in the safety of your own care. My parents owned a treasured anniversary clock received as a wedding gift. It had long occupied a prominent location on the mantle for all to admire. My recollections of Dad carefully taking the glass dome off to wind this beautiful clock are vivid. Fifty years passed. When I moved my parents to their retirement home, the clock was one of the first items carefully packed. The precious heirloom brought them great joy and Dad continued to wind it monthly.

Many years later, we would face yet another move. I knew the clock was key in making the new space feel like home. Consequently, on the dresser a beautiful domed clock was placed in a prominent position. No longer was there a desire to wind the clock, nor would it matter if it even ran. These things were not of importance now, but the symbol of what they represented was. This familiar clock was enjoyed until the day my dad walked by the dresser and in one swoop of his arm deliberately knocked it to the floor.

His caregiver, Tammy, relayed the terrible news to me: shattered pieces covering the room. She said Dad did not realize what he had done and was unaffected by the destruction. I found an odd sense of delight when Tammy told me that the irreparable pieces of clock had been put in the trash. The following evening, I carefully removed the dome from a family heirloom which occupied my mantel. The inexpensive imitation recently broken had been a clever imposter, apparently even fooling our dear longtime friend. I was certain my ingenuity would have made my parents proud.

Of course, room decor is just one aspect of these decisions; clothing will need to be carefully chosen as well. By this point in their lives, these folks have usually managed to hoard, I mean accumulate, an extensive wardrobe. I am aware all credibility for advice offered would be lost if my closet was on display. However, most closets in any type of retirement or memory care facility are minimal, at best. Simplifying is key.

Most importantly, choose comfortable clothing your loved one likes to wear, avoiding anything which cannot be easily washed. Elastic waists are helpful, as they facilitate dressing and bathroom routines, as well as accommodate for weight gain or loss. What we wear definitely affects our mood. If Mom has always worn dresses, now is not the time to start dressing her in pants. Likewise, if Dad liked to wear trousers and polos, don't dress him in loungewear just because his living situation has changed.

Consider the specific needs of your loved one. Are they normally cold? Then you will want to include more sweaters or jackets. A drawer full of scarves is crucial for a special woman I know who wears this fashion accessory daily. Likewise, cardigan sweaters occupy approximately one-third of my Dad's small closet. A small, basic wardrobe of favorite items, which make the individual feel distinctly special, is key. Two pairs of identical shoes will be helpful. Chances are, eventually a shoe will be misplaced. For the same reason, two pairs of eyeglasses are a good idea.

A wardrobe should be versatile; clothes which can be mixed or matched are ideal. If it is important for certain items to be worn together or you would be horrified to see your mother wearing her pink sweater with red pants, then it will be necessary for you to hang outfits together. The fewer wardrobe options brought, the better dressed and more organized your loved one will be. Keep in mind, clothes can be seasonally traded out as needed. Once you have chosen clothing for seven to ten days, label everything with a permanent marker or preprinted, iron on patches, which are inexpensive and readily available.

Jewelry is a more sensitive issue. Decisions involving wedding rings, especially, will be dependent on many risk factors. The monetary, as well as sentimental, value must be weighed against the joy wearing the ring brings. Ultimately, if jewelry is brought, the possibility of losing it must be accepted. There are a variety of scenarios, including a ring falling off due to weight loss, your loved one giving it away, or hiding it for safe keeping.

My mom was never without her wedding bands. They were a beautiful possession she cherished. So when my parents moved into their retirement home, I did not even consider taking them from her. Ultimately, they vanished. We suspected she had carefully wrapped them, for safe keeping, in tissue paper, as she had many other items. Drawers, as well as every hiding place we could imagine, were searched when my parents were out of the room.

Years later, as I packed the belongings of their apartment, I carefully sifted through everything, still hoping to find my mother's rings. Sadly, they were never found. Most likely the treasured jewelry was thrown away, either by an unsuspecting housekeeper or my mother herself. If I could turn back time, I would have switched the wedding bands out with one of Mom's pretty costume pieces or purchased something similar for her to enjoy. How I would love to see those rings again and have them to pass down to my daughters. They are truly irreplaceable.

Likewise, my dad had a beautiful designer watch he cherished and wore for many years. As his disease progressed, it was easy to replace it with one of the knockoff watches he acquired oversees. Dad wore his watch proudly on a daily basis. This proved to be a brilliant decision years later when he became extremely possessive of his watch. He refused to take it off for showers and became extremely agitated when the issue was pressed. It became the cleanest watch in town when I made the decision to abandon the issue and let him wear it in the shower.

Years before, my mom had faced similar decisions when packing her mother's belongings. Grandma's move became necessary when she began hosting large gatherings in her home. During one conversation, Grandma mentioned she had prepared brunch for several people that morning and was just cleaning up the kitchen. She went on to report the visitors were unruly, leaving her exhausted. My mother asked who these guests were and Grandma did not seem to know.

Alarm and suspicion grew, which prompted Mom to call a friend who was a member of Grandma's church, as well as the flower club she attended. "I have not been able to get Mary to join me in weeks," she said, "I've even offered to drive her." At first, some thought my grandma might not be feeling well, or perhaps age had simply slowed her down. This disease is adept at removing its victims from community. Ironically, the company of others is key in assuring their well-being.

Mom soon discovered Grandma had not entertained company at her house. She had been home alone and the guests she entertained were characters from her television. This dear woman had been overcome by hallucinations and overwhelmed by the demands they made on her. Unfortunately, this very real problem is not uncommon. For those with Alzheimer's or dementia, what happens on the television is often hard to distinguish from reality.

As you may have guessed, my final recommendation, albeit unpopular, is to leave the television behind. If your loved one has a favorite show, consider taping it without commercials. Arrange for it to be watched in the commons area, or with you. Viewing television in a group setting has the added benefit of socialization-interaction with real, live people. I have witnessed those with severe dementia have meaningful conversations while enjoying a musical on movie night at a memory care facility.

A beautiful replacement for the absence of a television in the room is music. My parents' collection of music includes big band, hymnals, musical classics, dance songs of the fifties, and other well-loved favorites. Just as one might turn on a favorite television show at a specific time, my parents looked forward to their afternoon tunes. Music can fill the room on a daily basis with pleasurable entertainment, which lifts the mood. An added bonus: it is conducive for movement, perhaps even a little dance.

"Because I have a name, make my room a reflection of the unique and wonderful person I am."

High Tide

*Joining our loved one's reality
as we learn new ways of communicating.*

We have reached a point where nothing can be taken for granted. What our loved ones can do today, they may not be able to do tomorrow. Learning to embrace their current abilities, while finding new ways to connect with them, is perhaps our most challenging task. Each day holds its own unique mystery, with few absolutes. As memories continue to be swept away by the tide, communication will become increasingly difficult. It is imperative to embrace this golden truth: every behavior is a form of communication.

To understand our loved ones, we must look for the reasons behind what they do. Those with dementia are not trying to be difficult, but rather attempting to express themselves in the only way they are now capable. Accepting there will be bad days and learning to approach them with humor will make life a little more manageable. Those experiencing the effects of dementia are doing the very best they can with the abilities they have. Knowing beauty waits in the good days and will grant us the strength, as well as much needed grace, required to survive difficult times.

130

Several years ago, I had been in a meeting most of the day. By the time I was able to check my phone, my parents' retirement community had left several messages, each more pressing than the previous. The predominant theme was there was a terrible problem and my mother, the beautiful woman I knew and loved, was the primary source. It became clear as I spoke to the facility on my way to the complex that Mom had set off the fire alarms.

Apparently, she was responsible for the evacuation of residents, as well as their subsequent stint in the parking lot. I believe I mentioned before; I loved this woman. Everyone knew she was mine. I was fairly certain there would be no denying this responsibility. I processed possible repercussions of the fire truck visit, a reality apparent from references made in an earlier conversation with the facility. This thought was fleeting; however, as images of my parents, being banned from their home never to be welcomed into another senior living facility, soon consumed my mind.

Much to my astonishment, I arrived to find my parents peacefully sitting in the commons area, holding hands. To the untrained eye, it seemed as if they were having an absolutely wonderful day. I joined them, secretly playing

131

sleuth, while attempting to gather pertinent facts. I casually asked about their day and they responded quite convincingly. If it had not been for the litany of messages on my phone, I would have been tempted to believe the accuracy of their report.

Finally, my mom, with eloquent speech and impressive vocabulary she had always been known for, said, "Well, I guess I should tell you about the shenanigans, because you will find out anyway!" "What have you been up to?" I asked. She looked at me proudly, "I have been directing emergency personnel all day." It was at this moment it became apparent more than just a single fire truck paid a visit that afternoon. "But luckily," she continued, "only approximately half of the facility was evacuated before I raised my hand and confessed!"

My mind raced with schemes of fleeing with my parents to spare them from condemnation. Surely the residents would resent this terrible transgression. How many people had been drug from their rooms and forced to stand outside in the heat of the day? This, only to subsequently witness a sweet smile come over Mom's face as she admitted to her "shenanigans"? I was searching for the nearest exit in which to make our escape when I heard a familiar voice. "Are you two sitting with us for dinner?" I looked up from my conspiracy to see my parents' neighbors. "Glad you stopped by," Dad said to me. "We need to go to dinner now."

I took my mom to the doctor the next morning and explained what had transpired. The doctor gently guided me through the day from Mom's perspective. We determined she had been on her way to the beauty shop and gotten lost. She apparently went up, instead of down, on the elevator. Once she arrived on an unfamiliar floor, she panicked. Not knowing what to do, the fire alarm offered a solution for her "emergency" and she simply followed its instructions. Walking through the events of the day in my mom's shoes allowed me a better understanding of an otherwise outrageous situation.

Her doctor then introduced me to the concept of good days and bad days. Admittedly an obvious proposition, but easily overlooked when one is in the midst of a crisis. "As long as we can agree this was a bad day," I relented. Disruptive behaviors are most usually the result of a fearful or angry patient. In my mom's case, she was scared and simply did not know how to remedy her situation or call for help. The unsettling experience was undoubtedly also responsible for her subsequent disruption in the beauty shop later that afternoon.

133

People with dementia often become confused or forget
how to appropriately express their feelings. Their world
is often a scary place where coping becomes increasingly
difficult. Pleading, attempting to reason, or punishing the
behavior is not effective. A person with dementia is
trying, to the best of their ability, with the capabilities
they have. Damage sustained to the brain makes
maneuvering through this confusing world a challenging
task. We only succeed at adding fuel to the fire and
keeping the issue alive when we offer explanations or
debate issues.

Imagine for a moment one of your most valued
possessions was stolen. Your wedding ring, car, or
perhaps a purse or wallet, containing a considerable
amount of money, was taken. There one moment, gone
the next. Obviously, you would be quite upset. Knowing
it has been stolen, what would you do next? Most of us,
undoubtedly, would reach out to someone we trust, in
search of assistance. Picture yourself in this position
and consider for a moment if these possible responses
would give you comfort and assurance your loss would be
recovered; the assailant apprehended.

Your most trusted friend, or perhaps the only person
you have a vague recollection of, is found. You explain,

through visible distress, that you have been robbed. This trusted soul flatly replies, "That didn't really happen." You know it happened. You experienced it. Your possession is gone. Why does this trusted friend, the only human being on earth you can find to help, not believe you? Why would anyone, let alone the confidant in whom you have entrusted your significant crisis, think you are lying?

You begin to cry. "It's okay," the supposed friend attempts to encourage. It most definitely is not okay! "This was very important to me and I want it back," you plead. Why is this uncaring person incapable of understanding how terrible the situation is? The "friend" realizes you are becoming increasingly agitated. Finally, assistance is offered. "I'll look for it," they say. "I'm sure it is here somewhere." You know it's not. You have already looked everywhere. Do they not realize you would not have asked for help had you thought it was here?

Exasperated, the unsuspecting participant further discounts your situation. "I'm sure you're overreacting," they say with the purest of motives. "Whoever took it undoubtedly means well." If we were to come across such a friend, no doubt a more helpful ally would aptly be sought out. Those with dementia live in a very small world where capable help is scarce. How frustrating it would be to constantly feel as though no one believed you. Sadly, I have personally witnessed, even found myself voicing, these ineffective and damaging statements, recited in an attempt to reason the problem away.

Although we are well aware the concern is not valid, it is just as real, every bit as traumatic, as if someone were to rob you today in the middle of a busy street. Alzheimer's patients often imagine important possessions have been stolen. If something cannot easily be found, suspicion is usually not far behind. The best response to this type of situation is, "How can I help?" Enter their world and acknowledge you heard and take the concern seriously. Above all, communication should be calm and reassuring. If the item is simply misplaced and can be found, then you have the opportunity to be cast as hero in this production.

However, something which cannot be found, or does not exist, will be a trickier proposition. In this case, redirection will be necessary. Often, a change of scenery is helpful. Going for a walk, or to the kitchen for ice cream, may help to focus on a new, more pleasant thought. Cookies and ice cream are proven remedies for all sorts of catastrophes. Depending on how progressed the disease is, an identical problem may resurface many times. Understanding and redirection are always key in alleviating the problem. Once a successful tactic has been found, it can usually be aptly repeatedly with predictable results.

Our loved one needs to know we are on their side, that we care and understand. Restating concerns by saying, "I know this is difficult," or "I understand you are upset," will calm our loved one's feelings of distress. There is no reason, nor is it effective, to attempt to persuade anyone not to feel as they do. Additionally, explaining details or the reasoning behind every situation or decision is not productive. Your role is to help; this is all any of us would be seeking. Simply relay this beautiful fact and repeat as necessary: I will help you; I will take care of everything.

Many times, you will find there is a trigger causing the distress to continually arise. My father's desk is one such example. When my parents moved to the retirement facility, I set up an office for my dad in the corner of the room. Working in an office had been routine for him the entirety of my life; it was an integral part of his being. Even though I had taken over all their financial matters, Dad enjoyed shuffling papers, sorting through mail, and making notes. It seemed like the perfect consolation for a man whose success had been so strongly attached to the symbol of his desk.

It was not long, however, until I realized this comfort was also a disruptive trigger. Not only did my dad's desk bring him immense satisfaction, it also was responsible for incredible anxiety and agitation. I began to dread the inevitable conversation which followed my parents' number appearing on my caller ID as calls became more frequent. "Someone has stolen my checkbook," he would relay. "I need you to take me to the bank and get this straightened out. There are bills I need to pay today!" Redirection only served to mitigate the problem temporarily and it would soon be back with a vengeance.

Reluctantly, I determined an experiment of removing the desk would be necessary in an attempt to alleviate the issue. The daily agitation had become so intense, I decided we had nothing to lose. While my parents were at lunch, I packed the contents of the desk and the maintenance staff helped me move it out. Either we would have a new, larger issue of a stolen desk, or I had stumbled on a brilliantly inspired solution. I did not know which it would be, but I was willing to take a gamble.

Surprisingly, my father never mentioned the desk, or his checkbook again. Not once after the trigger was removed did he communicate this distress. I had not realized how disruptive this seemingly thoughtful gesture had been. It only served to remind my dad of work which needed to be done and facilitate the frustration he experienced from not knowing how to accomplish it or what it was. Further, the desk highlighted a key element required in the process of completing the task. Sometimes objects trigger these unpleasant situations; at other times it is an unfortunate person bearing this burden.

Our familiar faces often serve as memories of days gone by, a past which is lost. Other times, an unsuspecting stranger may bear resemblance or possess a quality which initiates these feelings. An otherwise sweet woman at the retirement home became convinced her neighbor across the hall was stealing from her. She became increasingly upset, yelling at the poor woman on a daily basis. No matter how many times family and staff attempted to reason with her and ease her concerns, nothing seemed to help. She was convinced there was a thief which resided across the hall.

A brilliant resolution was eventually implemented. Although a move is not usually beneficial, in this case it was essential. After moving to another part of the building, this dear woman became complacent and pleasant again. No longer would she see the thief, as they would now be eating in different dining rooms and attending activities on opposite ends of the community. Perhaps this neighbor had reminded her of a devious individual in her past, or she may have just had the misfortune of being cast in this light. Whatever the case, sometimes triggers will not be alleviated with redirection and will need to be permanently removed.

In other instances, the trigger may be a figment of the imagination, one which may continue indefinitely, requiring some creativity to manage. Such an example would be the monkeys, which lived in the backyard of the house a woman resided in with her daughter and son-in-law. The woman was in a constant state of battle with her daughter, their main point of contention being the monkeys. The daughter apparently could not see them and became annoyed at her mother for constantly trying to convince her of their existence. Despite keen reasoning skills, the daughter could not persuade her mother the monkeys' existence was exclusively a product of her imagination.

Anger, frustration, and the slamming of doors became daily occurrences. Finally, the son-in-law stepped in and acknowledged the monkeys. "It sure is early for monkeys to be here," he said, "this isn't even monkey season!" He took his mother-in-law out on the patio to enjoy some fresh air and a cup of tea while observing the imaginary monkeys. The woman was delighted to finally have someone to discuss these interesting creatures with. She was finally allowed to verbalize her observations. The wise man encouraged her insight and listened with interest.

When they finished their tea, he suggested they bring the monkeys inside for the night, concerned it would be too cold for them outside. The woman wholeheartedly agreed. "Well," the son said, "they can't come inside without pants. Let's go inside and find them some pants they can wear." So they went inside and looked through a few drawers for suitable clothing. Soon thoughts were redirected. The issue of bringing the monkeys in was forgotten, but the lovely feeling the small investment of time produced remained.

Two of the most effective tools we possess in guiding our loved ones through frustrating moments are time and humor. The less of an issue we make of the problem, often the less of a problem it will be. Learn to find ways to incorporate humor into difficult situations. Laughter is a powerful mood lifter; everything does not have to be so serious. Above all, we should offer reassurance and respect in our efforts to relieve agitation.

The capacity to create a world of peaceful enjoyment will require effort and understanding. How terrible it would be if we were constantly being corrected. What a frustrating existence we would have if no one took us seriously. This is what dementia patients experience when their reality is discounted. Living a dementia patient's truth is not lying; they sincerely believe what they are experiencing. We must join their world because, the fact is, they cannot live in our reality.

My mom concerned herself with caring for everyone and always placed the needs of others above her own. This was a woman who went out of her way to ensure no one was ever offended, that feelings were never hurt. I remember occasions when I questioned a person's appearance, or someone's actions. My mother's predictable response was always full of grace and understanding. That is, until she was inflicted with Alzheimer's disease.

142

This sweet soul, who had maintained angelic perspectives, was also the voice which subsequently, and quite loudly I might add, made the following proclamation at a popular local deli: "There sure are a lot of ugly people in here today!" Do not even try to convince me no one heard her. Let me assure you, they did. Horrified heads turned and offended patrons stopped in their tracks, only to witness my dad nodding in agreement.

If I could have crawled under the table without making the scene even more horrific, I assure you, I would have. Believe me when I say it was thoroughly considered. My parents, unaware we were now viewed as adversaries, were presumably untouched by the glaring looks. These jolly folks continued to leisurely, blissfully, finish their lunch without a care in the world. Time has never ticked to a slower beat.

Several versions of a beautiful concept have been designed to aide caregivers of patients with dementia. These cards, the size of a business card, are discretely handed to those we encounter. The intention is to alert clerks, or anyone relating to your loved one, in hopes they can respond more appropriately. One of the more popular versions states: A person I am with has dementia and may have unusual behaviors. Please do not take offense. Thank you for your patience. Have a wonderful day! If only I had thought to bring a crate of those cards to the deli that day handing them out to the masses could have filled some time.

The fact is, the filter of a dementia patient quickly disappears. They will relate what they experience, often exuberantly, with an embarrassing lack of tact. It would have accomplished nothing to reprimand or correct my mom. She did not realize she had done anything wrong. Perhaps she had her fill of misplaced moles and wind-blown hair or, because of her habit of intensely staring at others, some less than favorable looks may have been shot her way. Whatever the case, from her perspective, she was simply offering an observation, such as, "The soup is extra hot today."

Communication, when experienced with a dementia patient, comes with a whole new set of rules. The most important truth to remember is there will not be a disagreement, ever, as long as you accept this one golden rule: They are always Right-Always-No matter what. We must stop correcting and erase the word "no" from our vocabulary. They are no longer capable of processing information as they once did. This disease is causing their brain to die.

Your loved one is not capable of changing. This leaves only one variable in the equation capable of changing, and that would be you. The simplest gestures mean so much to an individual who has lost so much control over their lives. When possible, create situations where they have some control. It is important to build our loved one's self esteem. For all our loved ones are no longer able to do, there is still so much they can do. Each one is a unique, wonderful human being with impressive gifts and abilities all their own.

"Because I have a name, remember everything I do is a form of communication."

Making New Footprints

*Seizing opportunities
to experience the adventure of life.*

After their car was "stolen" I planned frequent outings with Mom and Dad. We looked forward to our time together and finding activities which would give my parents pleasure was important to me. Taking on the responsibility of two individuals, who were still quite mobile and determined, was not easy. I made my fair share of mistakes during my rookie season of learning how to navigate life with my now unpredictable parents.

On one particular occasion, we went to the mall. I thought this would be an ideal outing with a variety of activities they would enjoy. We parked, made it inside the building, and continued up the tall, expansive escalator. A nail salon greeted us at the top, the location of our first stop, featuring pedicures for all. This was normally a mother-daughter date because Mom loved this special treat. Today, I brought Dad along hoping to introduce him to the fine art of trimming toenails.

He stopped short of the doorway, not as in ambling up, then hesitating for a moment. Stopped, as in a mule digging in its heels, then adamantly rejecting any further attempts to be moved another inch. Dad absolutely refused to enter. "That's a women's place!" he protested. Apparently, the male patrons sitting in oversized chairs with feet propped on tiny stools was not convincing enough. I conceded. I would trim his toenails myself when I took them home. "Okay, Dad, that's fine. You don't have to do this. We just need to go in and get Mom settled."

Obviously, I did not understand the concept of, "I am not moving my body through the threshold of this women's place." Luckily, Mom was familiar with the nail tech in the women's place, who happened to be a good friend of mine. She was graciously willing to come to the door, step over the threshold, and retrieve my mom. Dad and I spent the next five minutes walking a small corner of the mall, in an attempt to take in the other activities, I had planned. The remainder of the hour found us sitting on a bench an appropriate distance away from the door of the salon.

A semi-successful outing had been chalked up and I duly noted the obvious failures to be considered in the future. Down the escalator we would go and head home to enjoy a nap for all. Per usual, I followed my practice of getting on the escalator last when going up and first when going down. In reality, although I still believe this to be appropriate protocol, when reason is applied, how effectively would I be able to brace any fall should these two adults come crashing down on top of me? Nevertheless, this was the routine I had with my children, as well as their much larger grandparents. Mom held my hand as I retrieved her from beyond the threshold of the door; Dad followed as we made our way to the escalator.

I stepped on, then turned to guide Mom on. She suddenly, and quite unexpectedly, took a stance quite similar to one I had witnessed my father assume a short time before. Apparently, she had been taking notes. Feet firmly planted on solid ground, she braced herself, holding on to my hand with an intensity resembling clinging to a child dangling off a cliff. I had never known my mother to be a fan of baseball, but it is obvious in analyzing her posture she had observed and perfected the stance of an umpire. The problem was, obviously, my feet were on unstable ground, being propelled downwards on the moving staircase.

I believe the following events to have transpired over a period of seconds. However, this equates in real, "I'm experiencing this tragedy which may result in my death" time in slow motion. Realizing my mother was not letting go, nor would she be stepping on, I turned completely around and proceeded to run up the moving stairs. My feet searched for stability along the side of the escalator, then attempted to secure an open spot at the top. Mom had this real estate totally covered in her "I'm holding on for dear life" stance.

This brings me to an important point. Our loved ones are much more likely to cooperate when they do not feel rushed or forced into a situation. This particular event rendered, "Let go of my hand" and "I need a spot for my feet" totally ineffective requests. I distinctly recall specific expressions of passersby. Various looks of shock, concern, and horror were flashed in my direction. There was also a man who looked downright annoyed. Letting out an audible sigh, the bothered man shook his head before turning to disappear into the shadows of the store behind.

Everything happened so quickly, it is hard to put a timeframe on the events that transpired. What I do know is this: by the time I lunged myself onto the platform of the escalator, and tumbled onto the ground, clinging to Mom's legs, my father had completely disappeared. I suspect he felt as I had the day at the deli, and sought to distance himself from any relation to us. Subsequently, the assistance of security was required to locate him. As luck would have it, a security guard was among the bystanders now gathered at the top of the escalator.

I can only assume we come from resilient stock because, despite the challenges I experienced, I continued to facilitate meaningful excursions with my parents. Often, I would try to include them on small errands I was already running, especially those which they might find enjoyable. An opportunity arose to take my parents to the local wholesale club. I only had a few items to pick up and thought the store might spark their interest. After all, there were tasty samples available and the chance for exercise would be an added benefit.

We arrived at the superstore, I retrieved a cart, and they were off! Just inside the door, the enticement of two comfortable recliners beckoned. My parents took the bait. I wondered why the store had not included a big screen television in the display, just for good measure. This was not the expenditure of energy I had envisioned. "Let's go look around," I urged. "We will be right here!" my Dad convincingly replied. Try as I might, they were not budging. I mistakenly assumed this would be a guarantee of their presence remaining in this precise spot until I returned.

Despite my best attempts at racing through the store to collect the few necessities on my list, I returned to find two empty recliners bearing no trace of Mom and Dad. Apparently, moments after I was out of sight, my parents decided to look around. One's heart is never quite the same after experiencing the shock of a loved one vanishing. Adding to my distress was the fact that my lack of judgment was responsible for the predicament. Anyone who witnessed me that day could attest my pace, in frantic search of my parents, was even more frenzied than normal.

Luckily, the interesting displays and tasty samples inside the store kept their attention focused within the building. Soon after, I found them a few aisles over, gladly accepting an egg roll fresh from the slow cooker. Toddlers may move faster, but at least they can be scooped up and carried with us. When planning an outing with our much larger loved ones, we must realize the only power of persuasion we possess is of a psychological nature. Ultimately, it is imperative to be flexible, with their well-being our only agenda.

Although I would like to think I planned our outings wisely, there were times my best intentions were not enough. My nephew and I were visiting my parents one afternoon in a hotel room when they discovered we were on our way to the store. "We would like to go with you," they exclaimed, as my mom grabbed her purse filled with tissue wrapped treasures. "I would love to take you," I replied, "but we have a long list of things we need to get for the Academy and he needs them by tomorrow morning." "That's okay," Dad assured me, as he headed for the door.

How could I refuse my parents an outing? After all, I was responsible for their empty spot in the parking garage back home. If they became weary, or rather when... I would just have to manage the situation. "You know this is going to take a while, right, Dad? The store is across town and I won't be able to bring you back to the hotel until we are finished." "Sounds good!", he replied. As you may have guessed, I would not be relaying this story if all had gone smoothly.

One of my brother's sons, who I was raising at the time, had been accepted to a very prestigious high school military academy in another state. My parents had asked to accompany me out a few months after I tearfully left him to begin his studies, to attend his pinning ceremony. My mother, looking a very diseased version of herself and fresh from the battlefields of a diagnosis and traumatic move, pinned her oldest grandson as his grandfather proudly looked on.

My parents and I made the almost nine-hour trip fairly uneventfully. The only significant occurrence was a stop for gas along the way. I got out to pump the gas while my dad meticulously cleaned the windshield. Mom went inside to use the restroom. All seemed to go fairly smoothly, until the point in which the gas tank was full, windows were sparkling, and all had enjoyed a restroom break. I do not remember specifics, just that what I experienced resembled the task of herding chickens.

I was a bit frustrated, to say the least. After all, I did not have the benefit of Mom's, nor Dad's, driving skills by this time and this was a long haul. The enormous stack of photo albums I brought in an attempt to entertain my mother in the backseat fell terribly short. She constantly asked questions which demanded a response. The albums were simply not interactive enough to keep her attention. Finally, back in the car, we resumed the journey only to find the Interstate at a complete standstill a few miles down the road.

We sat motionless, burning the freshly purchased gas on zero miles to a gallon. If only these two would have cooperated, I thought. Why could they not help me out, just even a little bit? Dad commented on the unfamiliar body styles of nearby automobiles, as well as the fact several of them happened to be red. Mother talked incessantly; it seems she wanted to know what was wrong, again. I fumed.

There were events we needed to arrive for and clearly, this was not going to happen now. My best efforts at getting there on time had failed. I am sorry to say, I am quite certain the thought even crossed my mind: Why did I bring them along? Then it hit me hard—if it had not been for the delay, we very well might have been involved in the tragic accident which blocked our way. Since that day, I have never questioned a missed turn or traffic delay. Some things are just meant to be, perhaps even evidence of God's protection.

Eventually, we did arrive. As I reflect on the events of the weekend, I do not recall missing anything at all. We attended the President's dinner, had wonderful visits poolside at the hotel, toured the campus, and proudly snapped more than our fair share of pictures at the pinning. The weekend was winding down and I just needed to take my nephew to the store to stock up on necessities to see him through until my next visit. These traditional trips with him, as well as my daughters in college, are some of my fondest memories.

I had obliged my parents to accompany us to the store, in part, because leaving them at the hotel seemed more irresponsible than taking them with us-Even knowing we had much to do and could not give them our full attention. As I may have stated before, the store was across town from our hotel and by the time we arrived, my parents had lost much of their zeal for the outing. I may have experienced this before with my children, which had drawn my hesitation in the first place. We did not make it past the first item on our list before Dad announced he was ready to go.

My nephew and I were crouched on the floor with an assortment of credible sock choices surrounding us when I heard my father's conclusive proclamation. I glanced over my shoulder to reinforce my expectations for the outing when the large, lone frame looming over us took me by surprise. "Where's Mom?" I demanded. "Your mother is tired and ready to go," he informed me, "I left her on the bench." I should mention, my nephew somehow was not left without provisions. He did not hike barefoot at the Academy; I am reasonably certain of that.

The shopping list was abandoned in a pile of socks as we raced to the front of the store, only to find an empty bench. I notified the first employee I could find and a search ensued. After several frantic moments, Mom was found roaming the parking lot. By now I am sure a number of my readers have vowed never to leave their loved one, parents or otherwise, in my care. Regardless of the point in our lives this disease strikes our loved one, we learn through trial, error, and a considerable amount of mistakes as we go.

I share these stories, not to discourage you from outings, but rather to highlight the very real risk involved. It is important to facilitate enjoyable opportunities for our loved ones under our watchful eye. I soon realized taking both of my parents out would be easier with reinforcements. One of the more popular outings planned under this premise were Sunday night dinners with extended family. My daughters, Uncle Bill and Aunt June, as well as our dear neighbors, who were a surrogate aunt and uncle to my daughters, were regular attendees.

Meeting weekly, usually at the same restaurant, provided a familiar, comfortable atmosphere for my parents. They looked forward to seeing everyone and it gave our family and friends an easy opportunity to visit with my parents. These meals were reminiscent of our Sunday evening dinners of long ago. No longer would Dad and I walk the trails at the lake after dinner, walking to the car would require effort enough.

Dinner was routine, familiar, and comfortable. Mom and Dad's favorites were ordered weekly, which alleviated a confusing menu and the embarrassment of being unable to make a decision. After dinner they could always count on one of the girls getting them ice cream from the soft serve machine. I had the added bonus of fresh faces and helping hands when Mom inevitably required extensive coaxing to stand when it was time to leave.

It was at one such family dinner I first became acquainted with the art of joining a dementia patient's reality. Dad and I often discussed the outcome of his beloved college team's game at our weekly dinners. Luckily, his team was quite proficient at winning, which made for delightful Sunday evening conversations. This particular weekend, however, the team played horribly and had racked up a considerable loss. I dreaded the inevitable conversation.

Just as I expected, his first topic of discussion was the game. "Did you watch the game?" Oh, how I was dreading this. "Yes, Dad, I did." He squinted his eyes and continued. "What did you think?" I thought this was a conversation I did not want to have, that is what I really thought. "I am so sorry your team lost, Dad." Scooting back in his chair, he slapped his hands on the table. "Lost! What are you talking about? We won!"

It took some adjustment, but from that day on I allowed Dad to write the script. When dementia patients are allowed to dictate the realities of their world, we are free to simply join in. There is a beautiful truth I have discovered in this arrangement. The majority of the time, the script they write is a delightful one, usually much more pleasant than the realities of the world in which we live. "I am so pleased your team won, Dad!" An enormous grin swept over his face as he chuckled, "Me too," he said. "Me too!"

Surprisingly, some of my parents' most delightful outings were trips to the doctor's office. Soon after their diagnoses, I found an internist willing to take on both of my parents. This afforded them joint appointments which, of course, were longer but overall more efficient. Mom and Dad found many opportunities for mischief during these excursions. They were immensely entertained: doting on babies, mocking every cough and sneeze in the lobby, and inspecting examination room gadgets with curious hands.

Their antics often resembled lively toddlers in a china shop. On one occasion, Dad's aggressive observation ousted a container of empty vials off the wall and deposited them all over the floor. I can say with certainty this incident inspired the examination room's remodel. Luckily, their doctor was a kind and caring soul with a sense of humor. Regardless of what transpires at any appointment, medical or otherwise, the experience should always be followed up with a trip for ice cream.

The key is to find enjoyable activities that interest your loved one. Short, intentionally planned outings with extreme flexibility are key. Following our loved one's lead is imperative. My mom was much more content to stay at home, while Dad's on-the-go nature dictated the need for more stimulating activities. I often took him with me on outings while Mom stayed home with a caregiver. His energy levels and interest in outside activities was simply higher than hers.

A couple of Dad's favorite destinations were his nephew's body shop and monthly trips to a cousin's barber shop. One reason these visits were successful is the fact that, since they were related, the men Dad was visiting almost exclusively talked about the past. This was the connection they had, the historical stories they shared. The body shop, of course, afforded a delightful collection of automobiles in various stages of repair. I suspect the smell of grease and tires also sparked a chord of memory in my father's auto shop days of long ago.

Dad's barber grew peppers in front of his old fashioned barber shop. This garden was always of interest to dad, probably because gardening was his own mother's favorite pastime. As his hair was trimmed, Dad's cousin told family stories and inevitably ended on the note of how they were related due to their grandmothers being sisters. Dad would smile as he climbed out of the barber's chair, then inevitably reach in his pocket.

It is worth noting here that the importance of a crisp bill or two in Dad's pocket or Mom's purse never loses its importance. My father always had enough money in his pocket for the haircut, as well as extra to receive a bit of change. Tammy often took Dad on this outing, which was invariably followed by a stop for fried pies. Dad's treat. This simple gesture gave him a sense of pride in a world in which he had lost so much.

Outings do not have to be extravagant to be meaningful and, let's face it, we only have so many of those grand adventures in us! My parents' retirement community provided plenty of opportunities for entertainment. Monthly theme dinners were a favorite, providing pre-dinner appetizers and entertainment. Mom and Dad were always among the first on the dance floor when the band performed. There were meet your neighbor teas, bus tours, and weekly movie nights, complete with popcorn. The schedule of activities posted by the elevator resembled the social menu found on a cruise ship.

Shortly after moving in, a neighbor invited Mom to exercise class. Each evening before class a little reminder note was left under Mom's door. "I will be by in the morning at 9:45 to pick you up for exercise class!" This thrilled Mom and became an enjoyable activity she would not have otherwise joined. Also greatly anticipated were Mom's weekly trips to the beauty shop, otherwise known as social hour. Subsequent to this activity prompting her shenanigans, Dad began to walk over with her.

More than just a gallant gesture orchestrated by me, someone special was now living in a room across from the salon. This was a destination which Dad was eager to visit. The dear man who now occupied this room had been his steadfast friend since childhood. This lifetime buddy was a fellow boy scout as well as a groomsman in my parents' wedding. Pitchford, my father's affectionate childhood nickname for him, remained in Dad's life from hometown to retirement home. The sense of humor my dad and his friend presented could keep anyone fortunate enough to be in their presence entertained for hours. I am immensely grateful to be counted as such a person.

Over the years, Pitchford and his wife, Beverly, were among Mom and Dad's favorite companions on dinner dates and trips to the symphony. Soon after my parents' diagnoses, Pitchford lost his wife to cancer. I took Dad to their home to pay his condolences. This would be the most silent and solemn I had ever seen these two. In the months to come, Pitchford came to visit Dad in the apartment or treat him to lunch out. Despite my best efforts, I could not compete with this man. These excursions with his beloved friend were, hands-down, Dad's favorite outings. Pitchford was kind to take time for his failing friend.

He was responsible for carrying the conversation now while Dad played the role of a captivated, entertained audience. Occasionally Pitchford would call me to check on Dad or arrange a lunch. I received such a call one afternoon; one with a message I could not have anticipated. "I was diagnosed with a grand and glorious case of Parkinson's this morning," Pitchford relayed to me. "Could I come tour your folks' place?" It is so interesting to me, that over a decade later, I can recite, word for word, the exact sentence Dad's dear friend constructed to relay this information to me.

Ultimately, Pitchford moved into another section of my parents' retirement facility, which afforded him and Dad more frequent visits. This man held more secrets about my Dad's mischievous childhood than any other human being on Earth. He told unfathomable tales while Dad listened, wide-eyed and chuckling. I eagerly joined them to hear these dissertations every chance I got.

163

Lovely stories of Pitchford's wife were also shared. His room was filled with beautiful landscapes she painted on their travels. Each painting held in its composition a tale of a treasured memory. The eyes of the artist's husband danced as he relayed these stories. This dear man was usually found sitting in his recliner which faced the door. When we appeared in his doorway, an enormous grin inevitably swept over his face. "Roberty-Bob!" he would exclaim.

The first time I heard this endearing term, I was shocked. Undeniably tickled, yet shocked nonetheless. Apparently, since my father was not given a middle name, his closest friends had dubbed him with this legendary title. I found it unfortunate this little gem had not been brought to my attention earlier. This was just one of many secrets Pitchford held that my father conveniently failed to mention over the years. It was also one of many reasons I enjoyed these excursions to his room.

Unquestionably, these two were absolutely delightful and hands-down the orneriest any mother has ever known. There is no need for the adventures to stop when a diagnosis is received. Although the level of involvement and interest will change, there will always be something enjoyable to be found as you make new footprints. Now that responsibilities and worry have blissfully faded, there is much more time available for our loved ones to enjoy the simple pleasures of life. Make it a priority to facilitate meaningful experiences and continue to soak up the memories these moments afford.

"Because I have a name, please continue to fill my life with enjoyment and adventure."

Experiencing Sunsets

Embracing the realities of life,
as well as death, together.

Valentine's Day has always been one of my favorite
holidays. It is not the enormous boxes of chocolates,
roses wrapped in plastic sheaths and bundled by the
dozen, nor the mass produced red cards filled with
sentiments of love, which enchant me. What I find
charming are stories the day represents. This day
celebrates the promises we make when love is new; vows
we have every intention of keeping. It represents the
commitment of those who love each other well, weathering
the test of time and troubles.

Most beautiful are the stories of couples who are
fortunate enough to gather decades of memories. It is
unfathomable to me that two very different and unique
individuals could spend more years together than I have
been alive. Intimate years of loving and supporting one
another. Individual days of being companions,
confidants, and friends. Yet also the trials and
tribulation, which result in experiencing every emotion
known to man. A mutual life wrought with decisions,
challenges, change, and heartache, which emerges,
inevitably transformed. Memories collected together on

the other end of decades of life and love. My parents had such a love.

I found it so appropriate that their transition to the retirement home occurred on Valentine's Day. After being married over fifty years, this would be the day they were to embark on their newest adventure. A few days before the move, I began hanging pictures, filling cabinets with their most precious belongings, and placing towels in the bathroom. When the movers arrived the morning of February 14th, my parents had already bid farewell to their home of over forty years.

As the first piece of furniture was swiftly lifted on the truck, Mom and Dad were sipping coffee and eating brunch across town with Uncle Bill and Aunt June. Once the furniture was placed and final touches had been made in their new accommodations, my parents came home. I met them in the lobby and we all walked up together. Dad swung the door open, and to the surprise of all, reached down to swoop Mom into his arms, before toting her over the threshold.

After a quick glance around, they settled into their chairs and flipped on a favorite afternoon game show. "I'm sorry your parents aren't making a bigger deal out of all you've done," Aunt June consoled. "Their apartment looks beautiful and I know it was a tremendous amount of work!" "Thank you for taking them out today," I replied. "They are home and this is all that matters to me."

Mom and Dad settled into their new home and quickly learned to appreciate their lack of responsibility there. An aide came by in the mornings to administer medication, which was a much needed safety precaution. I called each day before lunch prompting them with the question of, "Are you getting ready to go down to the dining room to eat?" They managed well with this arrangement.

Dad enjoyed ordering meals from the daily options and Mom inevitably followed with, "Ditto." She was blissfully content, and unburdened with decisions, to eat anything her husband ordered. Life was frequently peaceful, orderly, and most importantly, safe. A new friend came three times a week for afternoon visits with Mom. This afforded Dad the freedom to attend activities in the commons area or accompany me on outings. This would be the routine for several months.

Eventually, Mom required more supervision. The biggest prompting for change came when she began to wander at night. A midnight call from the security guard, who relayed my mom had been found roaming the halls downstairs launched us into a new protocol. Furniture was rearranged to accommodate a second bed in their apartment, which provided for overnight caregivers. As time went by, each woman who was destined to care for my parents appeared at our door. Soon we had a team of four. Thankfully, eventually, my parents adapted to the new routine. Another book could be written here, but that is another story for another day.

These fresh faces provided Dad with endless opportunities for treasured practical jokes. Hiding was one of his favorite antics. The most usual hideouts were in the closet or behind the bed. A more successful refuge was on an obvious seat in the bathroom, which kept one frantic search on for several minutes.

Dad and I were leaving the building one afternoon when he spied a caregiver at the front desk. Her back was to us, and a cart filled with groceries beside her. All at once, my ornery companion swiped the cart and headed out the door. To his delight, he received an exuberant response. He turned to me and uttered these words, which I will never forget, "It's a good day!" Laughter is powerful, indeed, and has been the gauge in which I have measured my days ever since.

A more adventurous tactic Dad implemented was to lock caregivers out of the apartment when trips to the laundry were made. Adventurous, because this required Dad to get out of his chair, on his own accord. After one such trip to the laundry, a caregiver returned to find Dad's chair, as well as all of his usual hiding places, empty. Eventually, the search expanded outside the apartment and onto the grounds. Ultimately, enlisting the help of security was required. By the time I received a phone call, the search had been on for almost an hour. I frantically made my way to the complex.

Meanwhile, down the hall, Mrs. Anderson was in her bathroom getting ready for the day. When she emerged and turned the corner, a shocking surprise awaited her. Although she did not feel threatened, the large man curled up on her sofa was unusual, to say the least. The fact that he was napping with her cat, bizarre. This is amusing to me, only because my father was not fond of cats. (A horrible family tragedy involving a cat scarred us all, I am sorry to say.)

Not long after Tammy was added to complete the caregiver team, she went out on the patio one afternoon to clean the windows of my parents' second floor apartment. As she was making a final streak-free inspection to the sliding glass door, Dad suddenly appeared, peering at her through the crystal clear glass. He grinned, reached for the handle, then apparently changed his mind and returned to his chair. "How strange," Tammy thought.

After several minutes, she attempted to go inside and realized you-know-who had locked her out. This was of monumental hilarity to the man in the chair, as well as his giggling accomplice. Several minutes later, or perhaps hours from Tammy's perspective, my father recovered from his belly laugh. Rising from his throne, he cast himself as the hero of this production and unlocked the door. Mom enjoyed the fun for two these antics provided.

One morning several months later, giggles were heard from the bedroom as a caregiver put a pot of coffee on in the kitchen. Mom and Dad were accustomed to having a leisurely breakfast in their room. Often, they could be heard chatting as they greeted a new day together. This particular morning, Dad apparently relayed a comical quip, which spilled laughter all over their small apartment. In the kitchen, final breakfast preparations were being made before the process of rousing my parents from the comforts of their bed began.

Suddenly, a loud commotion broke out from beyond the door. Banging commenced as a lamp was knocked off the nightstand. The caregiver raced through the door of the bedroom just as a terrified, grey haired man sprang off the mattress and into the corner. She quickly led him to the other room and called the paramedics. Alzheimer's had revealed yet another inherent risk, leaving my mom with a broken arm, and the victim of a seizure. The ambulance raced her to the hospital for the beginning of a lengthy and heartbreaking process.

Although I took Dad to visit Mom in the hospital, being apart from each other was excruciatingly difficult. My parents adored one another; Mom could not pass by Dad without reaching for his hand or giving him a kiss. It was impossible to fathom them being apart. Everything possible was done to comfort my parents and make the process less frightening. One evening nurses at the hospital set up a table in Mom's room, complete with a white table cloth. Dinner for two was served bedside as two steadfast companions looked out over the beautiful lights of the city.

When the doctor finally released Mom, he informed me she would need to go to a skilled nursing rehabilitation center. There was such a facility in my parents' community and, thankfully, we were able to secure her a room there. From my experience, after the elderly have been hospitalized this is the normal procedure. This type of facility fills the role of providing physical therapy to help the patient regain strength and function. Most are located in nursing homes and are covered by Medicare. Unfortunately, these facilities are not usually equipped to adequately care for the needs of patients with dementia.

During Mom's stay, I often found her sitting alone in her room, with the call button in her hand. Many times she was in need of attention but, of course, did not know the purpose of the button she held, much less how to use it. I chose not to take Dad to her room there, but instead facilitated daily lunch dates in the dining room of their facility. Over the six-week period, the caregivers and I took Mom through the complex series of hallways connecting the buildings. My parents' mutual elation of seeing each other comforted my heart, which was ridden with guilt for separating them.

Thankfully, these weeks finally passed and Mom was able to go back to their apartment. Life returned to a new normal, a process which will be familiar to every family dealing with this disease. Mom would gain strength and improve, before faltering again. She made subsequent trips to the hospital over the next several months. Each time, upon her release, I was advised she would be sent to skilled nursing. Each time I refused. On one occasion, the doctor went so far as to tell me I was cheating. Knowing I had weighed her options, I defiantly defended the position I believed to be in her best interest.

I am not, in any way suggesting this stance for your loved one. What I am recommending is that you educate yourself on the options, benefits, and inherent risks of the situation your loved one will be placed in before making a decision. Ultimately, we have a voice in the direction of care for our loved ones. I do believe there is an urgent need for rehabilitation facilities equipped to handle the specific needs of dementia patients. In our unique situation, I concluded Mom's well-being was better served in the comforts of her home, where she would be in the presence of her beloved and under the watchful eye of their caregivers.

This experience prompted me to write a tribute to my parents the following Valentine's Day. Their resilience affected me deeply and taught me much about love. I came to realize love was not only a decision and commitment they made, which was tested by time. Love had become something integral to their very being, untouchable, even by this disease. A few months later, I made the decision to share this sentiment with family and friends at their retirement facility.

The air was crisp and fresh under the shade of the Oak tree. Daffodils were beginning to bloom and green blades of grass were poking through the barren, brown grass of winter. A new chapter of fresh beginnings was welcomed by the first signs of spring. The young couple sat on the stone bench, dreaming dreams and making promises. A year earlier they had agreed to double date with friends. Although they had attended high school together, they had not known each other well. The young man, tall and handsome, was back for the summer from a University on the East coast. The beautiful young woman was working her way through college in their Midwestern hometown. By the end of the summer, their love bloomed.

The quiet, sweet, articulate girl won over the charming, witty, young man. Sundays after church were spent getting to know her family and enjoying her mother's wonderful meals. He tested his skill at dominos under the old Pecan tree in the backyard with this beautiful woman's father and competitive brothers. She enjoyed long drives in this

175

endearing man's car, picnicking at the lake, and discussing the future. He determined he could not live without her and transferred to a nearby University the next semester. It wasn't long before they were dreaming dreams and making promises only the commitment and determination of love can keep.

Under the shade of the Oak tree he told her dreams of traveling the world. He promised to love her forever as they planned their wedding, a life together, discussed children, and the future. Hand in hand, they began their life together. Step by step, they walked their amazing journey, realizing dreams, and enduring disappointments. Grief never anticipated was shared; heartache no one could have imagined was experienced. Eventually, the young man kept one of his most fervent promises.

Together, over many years, they traveled the world, visiting every continent on Earth. This couple made lifelong friends and brought joy and humor to the lives of others. They made a difference in the world together.

A short drive away in the city, a confident elderly woman noticed a handsome, distinguished man, a resident of her retirement community. It was love at first sight. He, too, was taken by her undeniable qualities and soon they were inseparable. She was infatuated with his humor and good looks; he was taken with her determination and sweetness. She said he was funny; to the amusement of all, he called her feisty. Although the years stretched out behind them, their love was fresh and new. An enviable love only few find.

When she was stricken with health issues and they had to be apart, she visited him daily. As he noticed her coming up the corridor, his unsteady gait would transform to that of a sprinter. Arms outstretched, heart pounding, as if another moment could not pass without touching her. When he reached her, he held her, and told her he loved her. "Have you come to see me?" he asked. She smiled as if to say, "Of course I have, you're the love of my life." It was as if they had loved each other forever, and if the truth be known, they had.

For although life had brought them both joy and sorrow, rejoicing and disappointments, they had one constant. Through it all, the bond they shared was impenetrable. The disease which inflicted them both had stolen so much, the memories of their travels together, times shared with their children and grandchildren, the history they had together. It had even taken the knowledge of the promises made under the Oak tree when their love was young.

However, there was something even the devastation of Alzheimer's disease could not touch. The amazing connection between their souls was everlasting. Even through the confusion and theft of the memory of their life together, their bond remained strong. When she could no longer remember this man standing in front of her was her husband, the young man she married fifty-eight years ago, she simply fell in love with him all over again.

They slept peacefully in their recliners. The cold winter wind blew outside, but warmth surrounded them. Arms outstretched, their hands embraced the love of their beloved as they slept, peaceful and content. The two dreamed their dreams, certain in the end, they all would come true.

I patted Dad's leg and glanced at him through tear streaked eyes. He seemed to be fine, perhaps he had not realized this story was about him. Watching as the officiant left the podium, I put my arm around my daughter who was quietly sobbing next to me. My oldest daughter's voice now echoed from the podium, as she described my mom, "She was my best friend. She wanted to dance the last time I was with her. She got out of her wheelchair and danced with me for the longest time."

One by one, my mother's friends stood and expressed this woman's beautiful attributes. "Betty was so friendly; she was the first friend I made when I moved here." "She was a joy to be with; we went to exercise class together." "One of the sweetest women I have ever known." It was right to be here, I thought, surrounded by those my parents had lived with and loved these past four years. I was pleased this was the decision I had made. It definitely made the process more comfortable for Dad.

I glanced over my shoulder and spotted a man with suspenders; his wheelchair parked just inside the door. How good of them to bring him over, this precious man who had been my dad's buddy since childhood. His silent presence comforted me. Pitchford was familiar with this road we were now walking. He had survived the heartache. Perhaps Dad could too. I took a moment to acknowledge the fortitude we had been granted in the recent past.

It was just a few short days ago I found myself paralyzed, literally unable to move from the chair where I was sitting. I phoned the friend I found the first time I called for help, whose advice and knowledge of this disease carried me through some of the toughest decisions I have ever made. "I am not able to get up," I relayed to her, "and I will absolutely not ever be able to tell Dad what happened." My grieving heart assured me this chair, which guarded us from facing the realities of the future, would be my fate forever. "You will get up from that chair," she convincingly replied. "Your dad needs you."

What does this process even look like? I wondered out loud. How will I know how much he can handle? "Tell him what happened," she continued, "follow his lead and allow him to be part of whatever he wants to be." This is possibly the most insightful advice I have ever received. There are times I think about this day and continue to be amazed that I did, indeed, move past that debilitating moment. I continue to relish in all I would have missed had I stayed in that chair. I miss my beautiful mother every day but know my life, as well as Dad's, were destined to continue the process of living.

Eventually, I managed to take my friend's advice, roused myself from the chair, and numbly went through the motions of getting dressed and walking the next steps. It was Memorial Day. The retirement home hosted an annual celebratory spread of grilled hamburgers, hot dogs, and potato salad; everything one would need to appropriately welcome summer. "Could we eat in your apartment today?" I asked as we filled our plates. "Sure," Dad replied, reaching for a second dollop of baked beans. I knew I would not be able to eat, but placed an obligatory sampling on my plate nonetheless.

We went upstairs and sat at his table-my parents' table. I had given the caregiver the afternoon off so Dad and I could have some time alone. It was curious he had not asked about Mom since watching the ambulance dash her away a few days before. Of course, this was not the first time he witnessed such a scene. Eventually, she always came back. This time would be different; the horrible truth stung me to the core.

As Dad eagerly enjoyed his meal, I opened my mouth to recite what would soon change the reality of his world forever. "You know Mom was very sick when she went to the hospital," I heard my voice say. "Uh-huh," he replied. I briefly described for him the realities of what had transpired. "Betty, your wife, died." The finality of it hung in the air. It was as if my announcement had somehow brought this horrific truth to life, changing this man's life forever.

I honestly do not remember his response. The moment those words tumbled from my mouth, all strength followed. I am reasonably certain he understood, although the magnitude of the situation was undoubtedly impossible for him to grasp by this point in his disease. "She is at the funeral home, and if you would like to see her I can take you." He did want to see her. So together we began to walk through the unknown waters of saying goodbye.

After sitting quietly with me for several minutes at the funeral home and thoughtfully taking in the image of the woman he had so faithfully loved for decades, Dad announced he was ready to leave. One of the caregivers offered to take him home and lovingly stopped by the ice cream shop on the way. "I don't know who that beautiful, young woman was," Dad lamented as he gathered another bite on his spoon. "She must be a friend of Judy's." It is so interesting to me, after years of not uttering my name, he recalled it at that moment. So fitting that my mother would always be perceived as beautiful and young in his eyes. "Must be," our friend wisely replied.

The next day the minister came to my house to meet with Dad, my daughters, and me. We discussed our favorite memories, Mom's most beloved hymns, and the logistics of the following day. Dad made it through hearing the first sentence of the earliest memory before getting up from the table and walking to the window. As a result, he spent this particular beautiful summer morning on the back patio sipping tea and whistling tunes with one of my daughters. Although he may not have possessed the ability to fully comprehend the situation, my friend had been correct. He was still quite adept at determining how much he wanted to experience.

The following morning, we were picked up before the service and taken directly to the cemetery. I thought it best to have a quiet, family graveside before the service. The less interaction my father had with those grieving my mom's passing, the better, I thought. Dad and I sat in front of Mom's closed casket, surrounded by my daughters, and our closest family, including Uncle Bill, Aunt June, as well as the four women who had so faithfully cared for my parents over the years.

When the service was over, one of my daughters walked Dad back to the car. The other two consoled me as we bid farewell to our matriarch. I had not realized, as tears tumbled down my face, Dad could see me from his seat in the car. My daughter later told me a tear rolled down his cheek as he examined my sorrow. This was the only visible emotion he revealed that day.

As we continued our journey to the chapel of the retirement home, conversation filled the car. Suddenly, Dad leaned forward in his seat. Looking past two of my daughters, his focus honed inescapably on me. "What happened to her?" he questioned. Equally as piercing were the vigilant eyes of my daughters.

The driver glanced at me in the rearview mirror as the car fell silent. I leaned forward, looking directly into my father's ocean blue eyes. "She was very sick, Dad," I consoled, "and she died." I paused, then added, "She went peacefully." "Oh," he acknowledged as he leaned back and adjusted his gaze out the window.

I left Mom's memorial program by his chair after the funeral. Perhaps it helped to answer questions he was unable to articulate. Dad read the information and looked at Mom's picture often those first few days after her death. In the weeks to come we focused on planning a trip to the ocean to visit his sister. Dad would be living the reality of the absence of his beloved for the rest of his life. I saw no reason to force him under a cloud of mourning indefinitely. I could only hope he would process what he could, when he was able.

Soon after Mom's death, we visited the doctor's office for Dad's checkup and to ask his doctor's consent to take Dad on the trip. This was new territory for me, traveling alone with my father and navigating airports as a duo. The doctor thought it was a beautiful idea and granted his blessing, on one condition. "Get your dad some water shoes," he said. "I can't tell you how many of my patients have been stung by jelly fish." With a new sun hat and size 12 water shoes packed in his suitcase, Dad and I were ready to go.

The next morning, Tammy helped me get the last few necessities in his bag, explaining that I should display his toiletries on the bathroom cabinet as prompts. "In the morning, take the clothes you want him to wear that day and hang them in the bathroom," she said. "Turn the water on in the shower and make certain it is a comfortable temperature. Oh, and don't forget to lay the soap out for him!" This dear woman had facilitated my parents' care for so long now, I am quite sure she must have felt as if she was sending her son to camp for the first time. I eagerly soaked in her instructions as I apprehensively prepared to venture into this new dawn.

By this point in his disease, Dad was largely able to handle the morning logistics of getting ready on his own. With the appropriate prompts, it was reasonably assured he would emerge clean and freshly dressed. The most difficult obstacle of the trip, for which I was not prepared, was public restrooms. It was unsettling, to say the least, to send my father alone into a room I could not enter, one I had no means of retrieving him. I could only hope he would emerge safe and appropriately dressed.

On one layover at an airport, I found myself sitting on a bench at the entrance of the men's restroom, one heartbeat shy of a panic attack. Eventually, an unsuspecting, albeit reasonably safe looking, stranger entering the restroom was instructed to check on my father. If I had it to do again, I would have explored the location of family restrooms ahead of time. The same precautions should be taken for men with challenged capabilities as we would for our young boys.

However, these much older and larger male counterparts would definitely not be welcome in the women's restroom, as young boys are. Because I was in need of a restroom break as well, there had been that moment of opportunity for my dad to have walked out of the restroom. This question haunted me as I sat waiting, staking my hope on that bench with my eyes fixed on the men's restroom entrance. Thankfully, Dad and I arrived in sunny California and were equally warmed by his sister's glowing disposition.

Auntie greeted us at the airport with a handwritten sign scribbled on a large white board. She stood at the bottom of the escalator, donning a large straw hat and an enormous smile. One thing I can always count on when I see this dear aunt of mine: her eyes will be dancing in anticipation of our adventures. I cannot tell you what the sign said. Although I would venture to say each and every time we have greeted one another at airports, there has been a sign involved, the unspoken rule has been, no matter what the sign says, it will not be applicable.

Whether we retrieve a "Leisure Travels welcomes Mr. and Mrs. Waters" sign abandoned on a bench, long after the Waters are sunning on the beach, or handwritten "Welcome, if you're from Sam's side!" on a piece of cardboard, these memorable signs usher us into these rare and wonderful experiences we share. The laughter and adventure this week afforded the three of us was therapeutic. Auntie and I sat with Dad on stone benches for hours at the beach. Our faces shaded by hats; hearts comforted by the sound of the waves. We observed sea lions, enjoyed delicious meals at seaside restaurants, and delighted in stories of long ago recited by Auntie. On the final day of our trip, we all agreed it was time to venture into the water.

With Auntie on one side and me on the other, this precious man traipsed through the sand toward the ocean. Approximately halfway to our destination he stopped. "I need to take these off," he said, lifting a foot. "Oh, no, Dad. Leave your shoes on," I directed. We made it another hundred yards or so. "Stop right here! I need to take off my shoes." "Those are water shoes, Dad." My adamancy was defiant. His look was distrustful. We continued toward our goal.

We reached the water and anticipated the kiss of the very first salty splash as it prepared to greet us. My father reached for his shoe. "Dad! I promised the doctor you would wear those in the water!" "Oh, baloney!" my ever so compliant father replied. Moments later, the warm sand squished between his toes. Children ran by with sand buckets. Dad chuckled as he watched them splash in the water. A considerable wave lapped up onto his legs, dousing his shorts, as well as the water shoes he held in his hand. I could not resist. "Good thing those are waterproof!"

When we returned from our trip, the apartment had been tidied. Mom's clothes and personal belongings were quietly removed during our absence. Her childhood photos were replaced with some of Dad's earliest memories. The memorial program would not be displayed again. I was not attempting to erase her memory-this was neither practical nor possible.

What was achieved was a space in which Dad could resume his life without being chained to the tragedy of his loss. He was afforded some protection from having to constantly process her death. My parents' wedding picture remained on the wall, surrounded by photographs of other memorable moments in Dad's life. On the nightstand, a small engagement photo of his beautiful beloved would always remain.

"Because I have a name, please allow me to experience the joys, as well as the sorrows, of life."

Finding Treasure

Celebrating life with those we love
and being grateful for every moment.

By now, I had been walking this road many years and, although many had come beside me to help with the burden, I was largely on the journey alone. My daughters were almost grown, the youngest would be off to college in another state the following year. Apparently God thought it was time to bring this girl some help! My husband, Doug, is not only my partner and confidant, he has become the hand of my best friend who bravely and willingly signed up for this most difficult journey. He is the one I now turn to for advice and call on for reassurance.

Doug is the adventurous man who spontaneously drove me ten hours on a whim one weekend to see one of our favorite artists perform with the late great BB King. It was the weekend before our wedding. We did not have time, nor the money, for such things. We did it anyway. It would be our last opportunity to see this amazingly talented man perform before he was gone. Of course, we did not know that at the time, but it is further proof we must grab ahold of this life and live it with a passion.

Doug is more than willing to do this with me, so I gladly took his hand and accepted his proposal.

We were married in a nearby city, which posed a bit of a challenge for Dad. In reality, life is lived moment by moment now and, as my mother taught us, there will be good days and bad. We could have gotten married at Dad's retirement home and, if he had a bad day, an empty chair would have marked his place at the ceremony. Thankfully, Tammy and her wonderful man, as well as another dear caregiver and her husband were willing to tag team the journey up and back, as well as the evening's festivities.

When I began to walk up the aisle, I stopped on the back row to ask a favor. "Dad, would you walk me up the aisle?" With a small, encouraging nudge from behind, we were on our way. My father and I arrived at the front and my handsome husband-to-be walked down the steps to greet us. As Doug leaned in and shook Dad's hand, he said:

> *"Do you mind if I marry your girl?"*
> *"Well, yeah! That would be alright!"*

They laughed. I joined in, not knowing why this was funny. I kissed Dad on the cheek. With that, my father gave me some marital advice:

"Now kiss him!"

I duly followed his suggestion. As Doug and I walked up the steps to begin our lives as husband and wife, all eyes were on Dad. Tammy retrieved my father and guided him to his seat, now on the front row, beside her. Not a soul in the entire room took their eyes off of my dad until he was safely and comfortably seated. I know, I've watched the video.

Right about the time we were exchanging rings, our closest friends, dearest family members, as well as our beautiful newly formed brood of seven children tuned back to the event at hand. The one the invitation specifically mentioned would occur. That is okay. We all have grown accustomed to Dad stealing the show. He has always been a clever, comical man and this treasured sense of humor has only grown more enduring through the passage of time.

Something else has grown with time as well: the relationship between the two most important men in my life. My husband has become a treasured business partner for my father. Dad lights up when Doug walks through the door. I can visit my father all week long, exchange our usual pleasantries, whistle some tunes, and perhaps even get a kiss blown at me as I leave. But when Doug walks through the door on the weekend, Dad is ready to talk business. His gestures, voice, everything is transformed to that of one talking to a trusted associate.

You are not going to believe this, and that is okay. I would mightily struggle too, had I not been there to witness it myself. In fact, at one point I looked down at my legs, questioning if I was really there. Doug and I walked into Dad's room about a month ago to find him resting, which is not unusual nowadays. What was unusual is, when I kissed Dad on the cheek, he did not wake up. I checked to make sure he was breathing. He was. So I sat down in the guest chair, which was beside him, while Doug pulled the walker up and sat across from Dad.

Within a few minutes, my father opened his eyes to greet his guest. Doug. "Hi, Daddy!" I said. Nothing. He was quite engaged with the business for the day, speaking conversationally with Doug, although his speech was jumbled with a smattering of newly invented words. Regardless, it is a treasured gift at this point in the disease to witness him engaged conversationally. A couple of times he even gazed out the window as he talked, to Doug, conveniently looking right past me.

I am convinced Dad was not ignoring me, he was just that focused on his meeting with Doug. At one point my dad got exceptionally jumbled in speech and paused saying, "I'm sorry. I don't talk too good." Doug assured him it was okay; he didn't either. They both had a good laugh. I chuckled, but what does that matter? After approximately ten of the most invisible minutes of my life, I suddenly magically appeared in the room. Dad let out an audible gasp and said, (I quote) "How did you get in here?" Joining his reality, I told him I climbed through the window.

When we enter into conversation with a loved one with dementia, we should have the expectation of experiencing a beautiful moment. If we assume there is someone valuable waiting to be discovered, that is what we will often find. Conversely, if we think they have nothing to offer, that is exactly what we will receive. Rather than seeking to extract information with a series of questions, learn to simply experience their presence. Offer them treasures you possess: a warm smile, a compliment, a gentle touch.

The most rewarding visits are usually one on one, just you and your loved one. This is what made my invisible state so convenient, I suppose. It is amazing what insights might be shared with you, if you give them the opportunity. When more than one guest is present, the tendency for us to visit amongst ourselves is usually too compelling. Often the individual withdraws, finding it too difficult to keep up with the conversation.

The tendency to talk about a loved one with dementia, as if they are not in the room, is also far too common. Even at the doctor's office, the patient should be included as a valuable part of the conversation. Although they may be silent, they can still hear, feel, and are processing information internally. Their life is frustrating enough; we must guard against the indecency of talking about them as if they are not present. This can be extremely unnerving from my experience.

Limit distractions, shut the door, turn off the phone, and simply be present in the moment. Speak slowly and do not be afraid of silence. Conversation may come slowly, or not at all. When they do speak, listen! Be attentive and pretend to understand, even if what they are saying does not make sense. Everyone seeks to be understood; these beautiful human beings are no different. Talk to them. Even when they are no longer able to talk, their eyes will converse with you. Their eyes will tell you much about what they are understanding and what brings them pleasure.

Dementia patients like to hold things, whether it be a new handkerchief, a stuffed animal, a flower, photo, or small book. Bringing something to place in their hands is a thoughtful gesture that will illicit pleasure even when conversation is difficult. After finding the bucket of shells, I took them up to show Dad. He did not look through them, examining each one as you or I might do. What he did was hold them for a very long time. Eventually I persuaded him to help me put the shells back in the bucket, but I did not force it.

It is important to note that smaller items, such as shells, are not preferable. If they are holding something like this, do not leave them alone as they could be mistaken as candy. I can only imagine the host of memories these shells contained for Dad. He is no different than you or me, or the aide who exclaimed, "Shells!" when she realized these plain, white treasures were in the bucket I was holding. Grabbing one out she said, "Oh, I used to whistle shells, remember that?" I did not know anything about such things. Clearly, this was her memory. Finally finding one with a small hole in it, she joyfully celebrated her inspired memory.

Slow down, sit at eye level, make eye contact, and experience the emotions. Even when they are not speaking, they are feeling. A living human being is inside waiting to be experienced. Touch is a powerful communicator. It is a basic need from the moment we are born, and is essential to a person's well-being until the moment they die. A gentle touch on the shoulder as something important is being communicated, a hug while saying, "I love you", or holding their hand while telling a story all mean so much. Touch is also very reassuring and an expression of safety and care.

Offer simple suggestions, rather than complex choices, to avoid the frustration of decision making. Rather than an open-ended question like, "What would you like to do?" or a variety of seemingly thoughtful suggestions such as, "We could go outside, or watch a movie, or would you prefer that I read to you?" a simple suggestion, such as, "Would you like to go for a walk?" is a lovely gesture. They are then able to decide if the proposition sounds favorable and are spared from being bombarded by a litany of decisions.

My best advice in relating to Alzheimer's patients is to not quiz your loved one about what they can remember. Instead of asking, "What did you have for lunch?", it is better to say, "Did you have a good lunch?", if their lunch plate is still in front of them, or, "Are you having a good day?", if it is not. In this way a message of care and interest is conveyed without demanding the retrieval of past details they simply do not remember. A man with Alzheimer's once said, "Our value lies in what we are and who we have been, not in our ability to recite the ancient past."

Dementia patients are a product of their environment. If smiles and good moods surround them, there is a very good chance these qualities will eventually be displayed by them. Ninety percent of what they understand are not the words spoken, but rather the body language and tone of voice. Always be calm and respectful. Simplify the message. They do not need, nor can they process, a long, elaborate story with many details. Share a short, happy story with a dash of humor and repeat it as often as you like!

It is an adjustment, a conscious change in the way we view relationship with our loved ones. It is not easy. However, when we are able to enter into their world, we discover it is definitely worth the effort. These mysterious human beings are absolutely charming, often extremely comical, and endearing. There is still so much to be learned from them, so much to enjoy.

As his disease has progressed, I most often experience this when Dad and I are lost in a whistling concert. Although I have never thought of my dad as musically inclined, whistling has become a favorite pastime. This ability has been apparent throughout his disease process. On a good day, he is still able to pick up on a song after hearing just a couple of notes and whistle the whole tune quite impressively on his own.

Our concerts are most usually initiated with my three note introduction to a familiar tune. Three Blind Mice, Amazing Grace, Happy Birthday, and his alma mater's fight song are among his favorites. Dad joins in and continues the performance as a solo, usually completing the entire song with a powerful crescendo. My daughters and I are especially thankful he took the time to teach each of us to whistle many years ago. It is a gift which has afforded us the experience of many magical moments with him.

My youngest daughter was whistling with Dad last summer when a loud conversation outside his door took center stage. He immediately interrupted the concert and demanded that the interruption cease, shouting a less filtered version of "Please be quiet!" My daughter giggled at his exuberant reaction. He looked at her and responded, "We're busy!" Indeed, they were. This was a moment of great importance for both of them, which brought Dad immense joy. One my daughter will never forget. The concert continued, much to their mutual delight.

Sometimes my dad initiates concerts on his own, whistling a bit then expecting his visitor to duplicate the tune. Often the participant is graded according to Dad's interpretation of how they performed. His most usual classifications are "That's pretty good" and "That's no good." The most unfortunate contestants are those absent of a whistling ability, who are often met with a look of disgust. Truly, it is these unfortunate souls we should feel sorry for.

When we determine to experience those living with dementia as they are, rather than how we want them to be, we find their world is still very much intact. They are still relating, at any stage, as they experience and express life in their unique ways. It is a magical moment when we find that niche where we can immerse ourselves in their world for a few moments. With time and a little creativity, you will find an activity which affords you these beautiful moments.

We had an amazing moment of a different sort recently when Tammy and I accompanied Dad on a mandatory visit to the ice cream shop after his doctor's appointment. I find it so ironic his doctor's office moved a few years ago directly across the street from our local ice cream shop. If I didn't know better, I would think Dad had something to do with this. The challenges of the past decade have slowed my father down considerably and there is absolutely no way I could now manage an outing with him on my own. I am grateful for Tammy every single day.

After parking the car, I unbuckled my dad, then got out of the car. Tammy jumped out of the back and we converged at Dad's door. "Let's go get some ice cream," I said. He smiled. "Mr. Bob," Tammy cheerfully sung, "Will you come with us?" "Uh huh," he stated, in his now slow, methodical manner. So the painfully slow process began of persuading my father to lift and move his feet out of the car. Tammy and I then demonstrated to him how to accomplish the task once he was successfully convinced.

Over the period of several minutes we negotiated the process of getting my father out of the car and inside the building. "We better get in before the ice cream melts," is a helpful tactic, by the way. We continued our usual routine of Tammy getting Dad situated at the table while I placed the usual orders and got condiments. As I was filling the little white ketchup cups, a man approached me. He looked at me with tears in his eyes and said, "Thank you for taking care of Bob." I examined his face and was certain I did not know him. "Do you know my father?" I asked. He explained he did not.

"I saw you outside trying to get him out of the car, so I came out to help." The strong and capable middle-aged gentleman stated. "Once I got out there I was so taken aback at how you and your sister were talking to him; the dignity and respect you were showing him–it just made me want to stand back and observe," he said as he wiped away a tear.

I did not intend to tell him Tammy was not my sister–I will claim her any day. "I heard your sister call him Mr. Bob;

that is how I knew his name. I just stood there and watched you. I want you to know it warmed my heart and made my day. Your dad is a lucky man." I smiled at him and thanked him for taking the time to make my day as well. "We are the lucky ones," I said.

He then shared with me that his aunt was recently diagnosed with Alzheimer's disease. Truly, this epidemic seems to be touching every family. It is becoming increasingly difficult to find an individual who is not affected in some way. "She did not have children, so it is up to her nieces and nephews to take care of her," he relayed. With tears still forming in his eyes he explained he was the only one willing to visit her. "They say it is too depressing. I just don't understand it. She doesn't have a choice; she has to be there." We walked to the table together and I introduced him to my father and "sister".

I would like to thank the Glens of the world who step up every day to take care of their loved ones. *Thank you.* I am quite certain you do not hear those words often enough. I also know you very likely have family members who are not doing their fair share. It is easier said than done, but I would like to encourage you to resist the temptation to let this discourage or anger you. Also try to resist the urge to be resentful.

Whatever their reason for abandoning their responsibility, this is not your problem to bear. You have enough to concern yourself with to be worrying about them. Thankfully, dementia insures your loved one will live in the moment and is likely not bothered by the lack of companionship with these particular people.

Remember, you are the one with the amazing privilege of discovering this unique and wonderful human being. Sharing life with our loved ones is not over, there is much to experience and enjoy. You are the fortunate soul who will be left with the treasure box of memories. I guarantee this will be worth all the effort you have invested. Rich is your reward. Indeed, you have found the treasure.

Now, if I may be so bold, I would like to address these other people: relatives of Glen and the siblings of loved ones caring for their parent. Please do not take offense if you live out of state and miss your parents every day. Hear me when I say I am not speaking to those of you with unique situations. I do not pretend to know your family situation but have faith you will hear and know if these words ring true and are meant for you.

Over the years, I have, at times, thrown a private pity party for myself. Had I known you, I would have invited you, too, as I am sure you may feel deserving of one yourselves. The fact is, I have no living siblings. If I quit, my dad's world stops revolving. I have this immense responsibility and not just the lion's share of the obligations, but the entirety of them.

So many times I have wondered why, even been angry, over the fact that my brother "went and died on me", leaving all of this burden for me to bear on my own. I see this all the time and hear about it at every support group meeting I have ever attended. Children taking care of their parent, bearing the responsibilities, and the visits, and the decisions. The problem is, those voicing these concerns are not usually the sole surviving child of their parents-they have siblings.

So why are they carrying this load by themselves? Only you, the siblings who have thoughtfully pointed out concerns and details which need tended to so your brother or sister can put them in their bag of responsibilities, know why you do this. I am here to tell you, as someone who has done it on my own and only made it because of the help of pretend sisters like Tammy, your sibling needs some help. Step up and carry some of the load, or at the very least, reach in your pockets and hire someone who will.

The fact is, this isn't about us and it never will be. It is about someone who has loved you all your life and sacrificed to take care of you. This person now needs you to dig deep and find some compassion. They need the comfort of familiar folks and smiling faces. You are not familiar if they only see you once in a while. Unfortunately, what they are too often offered is an obligatory visit filled with expressions more closely resembling concern and sadness than the joy they would so eagerly welcome.

We are all confused about what has happened: uncomfortable in the present moment, and fearful of the future. But we are there, taking care of business, even if we fail to get it right. When you do visit, it is rushed, which is exactly opposite of what our loved one's need. When you speak quickly, our loved one cannot process the information. This takes time for those with dementia. Only if they are allowed to set the pace, can any of us appreciate life as they experience it.

Communication will drastically change during the disease process, which may leave our loved ones, as well as us, at a loss for words. Quite frankly, this stranger, offering only a faint resemblance of our loved one, is often difficult to converse with. Our own fears and thoughts of how unhappy we would be if we were in their situation, cloud the reality of what our loved ones are experiencing. Make no mistake-they will sense an uptight, uncomfortable guest.

I imagine, as children, by the time we have an awareness of our parents, we have already learned to love them. Or perhaps, just as I experienced with my own children, we love our parents instantaneously when we first lay eyes on them. Whatever the case, I had the distinct pleasure of falling in love with my parents all over again.

No longer were they able to do all the things they had done before. I would not be hearing how proud they were of me. Never again would I eat my mom's cooking or reap the benefit of my dad's advice. They had nothing left to offer me, yet they had everything. Regardless of whether they remembered my name, or even knew who I was. Whether they treated me with the social graces and appreciation others felt they owed me or not, they were mine. Delightfully mine.

I did the best I could to make the most of the moments we had together. Mom's death had taught me how fleeting these moments could be, even after a lengthy disease. A few months into walking through the unknown waters of life without Mom, summer was nearing an end. I had an idea for a day trip which I thought would provide an enjoyable outing. Possibly the change of scenery would be healing. Methodically, I began to plan this special event in Dad's nearby hometown.

Auntie spoke of some of these houses when we visited her earlier in the summer. I called and shared my idea with her; she was delighted. With her assistance, I pieced together a timeline of the dozen houses Dad's family lived in during his childhood. His sister researched locations and sent memorable stories. Armed with addresses and a GPS, Dad and I made the short drive to a small town only those who have lived there can pronounce. Once we arrived, we made our way to the first point of interest.

The self-guided tour began at the house where Dad was born. Dad was not a patient in a hospital until he was in his eighties! Conversely, the tour ended at the house where my parents lived when a wonderful surprise, fresh from the hospital, was brought home for their son's ninth birthday. Our tour took us down tree lined streets of his quaint hometown. I drove, ever so slowly, by every house Dad had once occupied. He was interested and definitely enjoyed the drive, although evidence of recognition was not apparent.

Many familiar sites were noted along the way. Among them were the high school, now housing the town's middle school, where two young men roamed the halls in search of mischief and brides-to-be. These beautiful women would eventually be found diligently studying. There was curious interest in an empty lot on the corner of Kansas and 4th Street downtown where the family car dealership once stood. A smile swept over my father's face as we pulled up to The First Christian Church and peered up the steps to the massive wooden door. This had been the door which was swung open all those years ago as Dad and his beloved wife took their first steps together.

We proceeded from there to the home Dad lived as a teenager. I paused in front to allow him a moment to observe the two story colonial red brick home. It had always been lovingly referred to as "The Big House", and aptly so. The home was grand in its day, sporting a parlor and dining room off the impressive entrance. A large kitchen graced the back of the house, with a large screened in porch, perfect for sipping tea on hot summer days. When guests were greeted at the front door, a

large swooping staircase welcomed them. The wooden
stairs, lined with a white pillar railing, elegantly ascended
to the ample bedrooms upstairs.

Dad and I were fortunate enough to tour the house many
years before, in a more impressive state. There was
something very special about the home, even now.
Suddenly, the previous resident insisted on getting out
of the car. What harm would it do to stand on the
sidewalk for a moment, I thought. Not that I had a choice.
Soon it became very clear my father was not interested
in merely standing, as one would expect a casual
spectator to do.

Before I could make my way around the car, he was
marching up the sidewalk. He then continued across the
lawn and made his way to stand front and center of the
parlor window, proudly taking in the image of the once
grand house. More than a coat of paint and the
replacement of splintered and missing columns would be
required to restore this home to its former beauty, I
thought. The current state of this beloved home did not
seem to faze Dad. He peered up to a second story
window above the parlor. "That was your bedroom," I
said. He smiled.

Soon he was, once again, purposefully traipsing through the lawn, as if he owned the place. Cowering beside him, I anxiously suggested we return to the car, certain the current inhabitants were relaying descriptions of us over the phone to authorities by now. Unaffected, dad continued, around the side of the property, past the screened in porch, and up a little rock pathway. There we came upon a stone bench, the setting for promises and precious moments during my parents' courtship. Dad stopped and took a long, deep breath, as if he was retrieving a memory of long ago.

I soaked in images of moments of long ago as well, and acknowledged how pristine this setting once was. Random flowerbeds, now wild and unkept, hosted daylilies and phlox, to the delight of numerous butterflies. They fluttered and danced, celebrating this beautiful late summer day. My father paused under the shade of the Oak tree as streaks of sunlight made their way through its boughs. He stooped down, placed his hand on the bench, then took a seat. I smiled, then joined him, having long since forgotten we were, technically, trespassing.

A yellow butterfly fluttered by, then danced around us. It was such a beautiful day; I was so glad we had come. I looked at Dad and placed my hand on his knee. He smiled as the dancer lit on his shoulder. Time stood still. This was one of the most amazing moments I have ever known. We sat for some time-my father, the dancer, and I. Never had the ambiance of an unknown place felt so familiar. The look of pleasure on Dad's face taught me something significant that day-although memories cannot be forced, they can certainly be inspired.

It seemed as if we spent decades soaking in the memories this beautiful setting offered. Then with a deep, contented sigh, my father stood. As we continued up the rocky trail, his gaze lifted as he thoughtfully took in the image of the now somewhat dilapidated garage. The second floor of this structure housed a small apartment-my parent's first home as newlyweds.

I considered how many storms this garage apartment had endured, yet strongly stood the test of time. How many unspoken secrets it now held of its vibrant history? Not unlike my father, I thought. I put my arm around this faithful promise maker. "It's beautiful," I whispered.

"Because I have a name, please join my world where we can share sweet moments together."

Crashing Waves

Embracing with compassion what we cannot change.
Fighting with fervency that which we must.

These waters are treacherous, at best. Although it is often painfully difficult to keep our heads above water as the waves crash in on us, it must be exponentially harder for our loved ones. They are in desperate need of our reassurance. "I understand," or "I would feel the same way, too," are beautiful gestures which offer the understanding they are seeking. Short, simple answers are best. When we elaborate with longer responses, we are often met with confusion or intense debate.

A loving tone and reassuring body language open the door for more positive communication. If all else fails, ice cream is a magical word, universally recognized with impressive results. I have unfortunately expended vast amounts of energy in a quest for my dad's compliance, only to have him forget what he has agreed to do. This was quite possibly one of the most difficult lessons I had to learn. I wanted to relate to Dad in the only way I knew.

My father and I always had a wonderful relationship. (For the most part, when he wasn't tossing me out and slamming the door behind me.) He teased me as a teenager when I left the house: "Don't let the doorknob hit you in the back on your way out!" Mom warned him urgently and often he was going to hurt my feelings. He didn't. I knew. This is why the sticky note on my bathroom mirror on my 18th birthday was so funny.

"Happy Birthday, Sweetheart! Don't let the doorknob hit you on the back on your way out!"

Mom would have been horrified if she knew. Luckily, she was occupied arranging my perfectly wrapped gifts on the breakfast table. She was equally as amazing as my dad. He was my confidant, advisor, friend, and walking buddy, as well as one of my biggest cheerleaders. From the moment we learned of his disease, my desire was to help him understand. My attempts to convince that certain decisions had to be made left us both feeling frustrated and defeated.

He was not capable of rationalizing these decisions. The more fervently I presented these propositions, the more fiercely he opposed them. I began to see the wisdom in protecting him from the heartache of difficult absolutes. Slowly I learned to implement decisions without looking to him for the approval I was never going to receive. He was no longer the competent father I had known all my life. The time had come which we had

213

outlined years before. I had to step into the role I agreed to take on should he ever become unqualified to make reasonable decisions. It was my job to protect him, sometimes from himself.

The best advice I ever received was from my friend, Paula Avery: "Do not try to negotiate or reason with a dementia patient." Our loved ones inflicted with dementia have lost the ability to rationalize. Communication often becomes an exercise in psychology. This requires creativity. What is effective today may not work tomorrow, so we must stay intuitive and flexible. It is magical when a solution is discovered that effectively alleviates the problem. However, be prepared for the progression of the disease to eventually dictate change.

It is extremely unusual for anything to work forever, with the exception of ice cream and cookies, of course. My dad's proximity to his childhood friend had also afforded a delightful outlet of laughter and many wonderful visits. I was thankful he had the gift of this friendship. Many times over the years, Tammy or I walked Dad over to meet in Pitchford's room or sit with him for lunch. It was amazing to me that my father could always spot his friend from across the room.

On one occasion, Dad pointed through a crowd of people, to the back of a grey-haired man who was sitting at a table across the room. "There he is!" Dad exclaimed, redirecting his steps towards the man. I was convinced this was not Pitchford. I tried fervently to convince Dad so this escapade would not end in embarrassment. He would not listen. Come to find out, I was wrong.

After Mom's death, it was important to me for Dad and his buddy to get together. I knew Pitchford would provide a source of connection and meaning to my father's life. One day, I encouraged Dad to walk over to his room. "Would you like to go with me to visit Pitchford?" He looked at me in bewilderment. "Who?" I stated Pitchford's first name a few times, in a progressively louder voice. And it is just now occurring to me- why do we do this? My Dad is not even the slightest bit hearing impaired. He simply cannot understand the question being posed.

I stated Pitchford's full name, as if I were calling him to the stand for testimony. I then stated with the utmost authority, "Pitchford, your buddy." I searched for a glimmer of recollection in Dad's eyes and found none. "I don't know who that is," he said. "That's okay," I responded. "I am headed down to get some cookies. Would you like to come?" He did. Once downstairs, I victoriously redirected him away from the bench which grandly welcomed us as the elevator doors opened.

Tammy taught me everything I know on the finer points of this tactic. I quite impressively played blocker that day between my father and the seat he inevitably would have taken if given half a chance. I was grateful Tammy had accumulated vast amounts of expertise on the matter. She would be proud of my performance. This bench, which was just outside the elevator doors, had been the location of a meeting spot years ago when Pitchford came to take his friend, recently deprived of a car, out to lunch.

They met often over the course of their friendship, which now spanned over seventy-five years. As luck would have it, in their younger days, Pitchford's office was located across the street from one of my father's apartment complexes. Dad's first job in the city selling investments eventually led to opportunities investing in apartments. His dream was to buy his own complex. Eventually, Dad's dream came true in the purchase of a run-down complex in a forgotten part of town.

This would be my first job-cleaning the furnished apartments. The scent of Pledge is vivid in my mind.

My dad walked me to the next apartment needing a good cleaning before it was ready to rent and set a time to pick me up. A quick text on the cell phone when I was finished would have been handy, but unfortunately was unavailable at the time. "Lock the door," he inevitably said. I always did. I was not allowed to walk the parking lot alone. After all, the manager, Mrs. Hulsey, had been robbed at gunpoint more than once.

Any trip back to our hometown to visit both sets of my grandparents always included a "quick swing by" the apartments to check on whatever it was that always, without doubt, had to be attended to in the manager's office. Mom and I stayed safely in the car under the watchful eye of my vigilant brother, who would have been listening to Rock-n-Roll on his IPhone, had it been invented. I often wondered what was so important that this delay to Grandma's was so necessary. I have since found out.

My dad was the apartment owner and beloved landlord who could be found in his blue jeans and cowboy boots, alongside his maintenance man, moving refrigerators, fixing disposals on Thanksgiving Day and rushing away from Christmas dinner to investigate a burst water pipe. He was the kind and generous boss who was committed to a better life for his employees and treated each one like family. Eventually, as fate would have it, the forgotten neighborhood burned down a good portion of Dad's apartment complex and the city demanded he call in a demolition crew.

Covered in soot yet not defeated, my Dad fixed his goal on a complex close to our home. Since he had been "pinching pennies" for some time, he decided to buy it. Dad marched up to the door of the elderly couple who owned the complex (which happened to be on the same property the house in question was located) and kindly told the man he would like to buy the place. I am fairly certain this type of arrangement was taught to him by my grandfather. I could have told Dad this would not have a good outcome. I knew. I had tried such a tactic of Granddad's. The door was slammed in his face.

I have only seen this expression on my father's face three times, that I can recall. When he relayed to us over dinner that night, "He slammed the door in my face!" (The face my father was referring to would be the face of its future owner.) The second was when my parents relayed to me that my brother had been murdered, and the third when my father received his diagnosis. It is interesting to me that Dad's expression was identical each time, his tenacity equally matched. However, somehow, each time the ability to fight had become increasingly diminished.

Dad walked over at least once a week to meet Pitchford for lunch at a picnic table by a pretty little creek that ran through the property of the telephone company where this childhood buddy worked. Sometimes the ducks on the pond of the property (the one which was finally victoriously purchased with pinched pennies) followed the owner over to hear tales of his childhood. There were countless experiences these two friends shared through the years. I looked forward to hearing which gem from his memory bank Pitchford would relay today.

Perhaps I failed to mention that I had every intention of walking over to Pitchford's room, as soon as we gathered some cookies from the tray. I had not mentioned it to my father either. We arrived to find Pitchford, predictably, in his recliner. He wore a large bandage on his head, the result of a tumble over the rubber strip in the threshold of his bathroom door. He looked up as we entered his room. "Roberty-Bob!" he exclaimed, "Did you bring me any money?" A smile came over Dad's face, "The bank is closed, Pitchford!"

The instant he saw his friend, a memory was rekindled and scripts from the past were recited. I was hoping they would be. How I treasured these glimmers of the father I had known. Our favorite storyteller would not make us wait long for a tale. Pitchford chose one of his favorite characters to cast in the production today; a young boy from the childhood of two ornery boys. A fellow boy scout, who seemed destined for misfortune. I had formed vivid images of this lanky lad from the glorious tales these men, the best friends inhabiting the current stage before me, had told of him over the years.

One such story, taking place in a variety of locations over a considerable period time, found their unusual friend constructing wings out of a variety of materials. The boy ran off ramps, jumped off diving boards, and even catapulted himself off the roof of a car in an attempt to test his theory. At least this is how the story was told. I chose to believe every word. Apparently, he eventually constructed some wings that met his exacting standards. Curiously, my current companions were always cast in the wings of these productions as innocent bystanders, curtain crew, presumably silently in the shadows.

Of course, I knew better, but never attempted to challenge the script. Ultimately, the misguided lad strapped these enormous wings on his back, while apparently two quiet and curious onlookers casually observed. This is where, unfortunately, the tale gets unbelievable. (Believe what you will, I am simply relaying the facts as I know them.) After climbing onto the roof of the house, fate and science were soon to be tempted. How old was this boy, I wondered? How I wish I could ask this and many, many more questions.

Despite this young man's ardent attempts, he soon discovered this particular set of wings failed to equip him to fly. This, unfortunately, resulted in a tumble off the roof of his house, as well as a broken arm. Pitchford was clever and I would be tempted to think he had recently written this script, had it not been for my father's reaction. Pitchford's storytelling, I mean reporting of facts, of course, was vivid, but something more was tapped into in order to achieve the response I inevitably witnessed in my father.

This particular day we were to hear a campfire story. The fact that my dad was one of the characters cast made these tales absolutely delightful. "We had some adventurous campouts when we were boy scouts,"

Pitchford recollected. Fortunately, their unfortunate friend was also cast in most of these childhood stories, which assured the present audience of a fabulous tale. "He just never seemed to be able to get anything right," the childhood buddy continued. Dad sat in eager anticipation.

"Remember the time he was trying to warm that can of beans over the campfire?" Pitchford rhetorically asked. Of course, I had not been there and these memories had long since been swept away in the tide of Dad's disease. "Everyone knows you have to take the lid off first!" Pitchford chuckled and Dad followed suit, clearly pleased to hear the story.

Attempting to gain his composure, Dad's buddy geared up for the punch line. "Those beans exploded all over us!" It seemed as if he could hardly breath as he heartily laughed. Dad was gasping for air as well, as his whole body shook with enthusiastic laughter. I giggled as well, but this moment was not about me.

"We were covered in beans!" Pitchford relayed, as he wiped tears of laughter from his cheeks. "There were burns all over our arms!" he took a deep breath and smiled at my father, "Do you remember that, Roberty

Bob?" Dad looked at his friend, wide-eyed, soaking in the story. If only he could make images out of the words spoken, perhaps the incident could be retrieved out of the crevasses of his memory. Dad chuckled at the hilarity of Pitchford's recollection. I tucked one more precious story about my dad and his friend into my basket of shells.

Our dear friend's health continued to decline in the months to come. Parkinson's disease continued to wreak havoc on his motor skills, thanks to the death of vital nerve cells in his brain. This chronic and progressive dementia was the root cause of many falls. Tammy took Dad, one last time, over to see him. (Not that we ever know when that moment is occurring.) Pitchford was in bed and not very responsive. It was apparent how painfully difficult it was for my father to see him this way. Because my father no longer remembered him until he saw his image, we made the decision to no longer facilitate these visits.

A few weeks later, Tammy called me to relay that Pitchford was being moved to a hospice facility; they would be coming that day. "He is not doing well, Judy." I asked when he would be moved so I could be there before hospice came to get our friend. This dear man has to be scared, I thought. Pitchford and Beverly did not have any children, and although he had close friends that oversaw his care, I considered him family.

I thought about these precious memories as I drove to see this man who had been a part of my life since childhood. With the move to another facility, I knew our visits would be sparse. A lone, wet tear rolled out of the corner of my eye as I realized my father would, in all probability, never see his friend again. The stories would cease. I remembered years ago, after the death of one of Dad's friends, he said, "All my friends are dying! I only have Pitchford and a few others left!"

My heart was constructing things to say to him today. He needed to know how much he meant to us all and how much we loved him. I wanted him to understand how I treasured his stories and the gift those laughter-filled visits were. Perhaps they needed help packing Beverly's paintings. How I hoped someone would take the time to hang a few in the hospice room. He would need that comfort in the days to come. I gathered my thoughts and offers of encouragement and walked through the door of his building for what would be the next to last time.

When I arrived at his room I prepared myself for his now frail body. Tammy had warned me he had gone down quickly. I did not have much to offer him, but I hoped my presence and hand to hold would give him comfort. Each time I had visited him, I asked him to call me if he needed anything. He never did. Perhaps he would now. I turned the corner only to find an empty bed, stripped of sheets. The halls were vacant of aides, so I hurried to the receptionist's desk. Why had they moved him so soon?

I needed to find out which hospice he was taken to so I could help him get settled in. I reached the desk and frantically relayed my question to the receptionist. She, in turn, relayed an answer I did not wish to receive. It was too late. Before the plans of hospice were carried out, Pitchford quietly joined Beverly, just beyond the sunset. I clung to my jagged rock and assessed the damage of yet another passing. The sun set on another day, one with challenges and heartache. A day which had not gone as planned.

Life took my calendar, rearranged the events, and ripped out another page, tossing it in the water. My father and I would once again watch the sun rise on a new day and attempt to find our way down the rocky shore. We were called on to navigate death too many times. My brother's murder threatened to rip us apart as it sent the three of us running to our own grief-stricken corners. We licked our wounds and tried to make sense of this tragedy, each in our own way. Meanwhile, the hands of time kept ticking, propelling us into an uncertain future. When my brother was horrifically murdered, a little piece of my parents and I, as well as his sons, died.

My brother's body was never found.

We came crawling out across the rocky shores of this tragedy, scarcely catching our breath before the next round of crashing waves dealt us the blow of Mom's diagnosis.

The waves violently swept my mother out to sea.

As I was attempting to piece together the realities of this unimaginable blow, another relentless wave crashed.

And Dad was swept away by the current.

All I could do was to stand on the shore, waving my arms frantically in the air, and screaming at the top of my lungs in a language now unfamiliar to them, "Get out!! There's danger in the water!" If only they could have reached the shore. I had no choice but to swim into the ghastly horror, filled with the blood of its victims, the anguish of their pain.

Five years after Mom's death, I was still trying to make sense of a life absent of her presence. Dad and I were attempting to walk down the beach, in the murky tide soaked sand, trying to catch our breath before the next wave swept us away. We no longer walked with confident strides. We were too beaten down to do anything but pick up one foot at a time and hope somehow when we put it down it would be heading somewhat in a reasonable direction.

With that, another disease of dementia took Pitchford's life.

There was a simple notice in the paper. Mr. Pitchford passed away. Just like a whisper, this man walked into one of Beverly's beautiful paintings and disappeared. His best buddy did not even shed a tear. He couldn't, for he would never be told. My heart grieved like a violent, terrible hurricane which would not let me go, as I imagined telling my father of Pitchford's death only to hear him respond with, "Who?" I was going to have to go this one alone. I wiped my tears, and grabbed Dad's hand as we picked up another foot.

Yet another sweeping wave of change was just around the corner, hiding in the distance. Just beyond the next bend, Dad and I found ourselves at an impasse we could not cross. We were going to have to get in. I was terrified. Clearly, my father did not understand-he couldn't. The same disease which took my father's best buddy had now struck him. His doctor compassionately delivered the news.

"You have Parkinson's disease."

This time there would be no utterance of, "It *is* happening to someone! It's happening to *me*!" Nor did my father say, "Wouldn't it be just awful if that happened to someone?" He simply sat, hands quietly folded, head down, taking intermittent rests as his tremors shook the capable, strong hands of my father, rendering them uncontrollably stricken with another cruel disease of dementia.

How relentless this thief had been to us, I thought. Why did it have to strike our family, not only once, but twice, before it continued to crash in on us relentlessly, slamming us into the jagged rocks of despair? Another tear rolled down my face. I honestly did not know how much more I could take. The waves were pulling me under. I could not hold on much longer and I knew we were not ever escaping this storm.

My father looked up and turned his gaze on me. I drew a smile out of the deepest crevasse of my soul. He smiled back, one of his tiny, closed mouth crooked smiles and whistled. This demanded my mimic and I had better do it well. I knew I would be graded. I drew a deep breath and gave it my best performance. My father had no choice, he was on the train and it was headed for an inescapable destination. Knowing he would not survive without me, I chose to buy a ticket too.

Two months before I moved my father to Memory Care, I received a call from Aunt June. "Judy, your Uncle Bill went to the post office this morning and never came home." Ironically, I was at the salon sitting with the friend who had graciously walked my mom over the threshold of the woman's place more than a decade ago. "I'm so sorry," I said as I leaped from the chair, "I have to go!" My friend raced after me. When she finally caught up, I heard her whisper in my ear:

"I am going with you!"

After retrieving Aunt June, we arrived at the hospital to begin our wait while stints were placed in my uncle's heart. Doug arrived and took the precious friend who had held my hand to the gas station where they would retrieve my uncle's car. Uncle Bill had collapsed in the parking lot due to a heart attack. Had two compassionate and caring individuals not rendered CPR that day, we would have been experiencing yet another death.

Uncle Bill spent the following days recuperating and telling his grand tale of a life miraculously spared. Both of his rescuers visited him in the hospital on more than one occasion. All three of my daughters came to see this fortunate man, hug his neck, and tell him how much he was loved. Most importantly, Aunt June spent precious moments by his side. Eventually, he was moved to skilled nursing to recuperate. My aunt and I began the process of touring facilities in an attempt to find a new home for them when he was released.

They would need assisted living, at the very least. Obviously, Uncle Bill could no longer manage life, as they knew it, in their home. Aunt June was going to need some help. I passed through the same doors when Pitchford died. Little did I know this would be my final visit with my uncle as well. Uncle Bill was soon taken back to the hospital; his vitals were not good. We raced back to be by Aunt June's side. When we arrived at the hospital, we were told the news. Less than three weeks after the morning Uncle Bill got in his car and drove away, we realized he would not be coming back at all.

Uncle Bill died of pancreatic cancer.

Parkinson's disease took Dad down physically very quickly. As a result, he made his first appearance as a patient at the hospital when he was eighty-two years old. Dad had become unstable. When he stood, he seemed to be quite dizzy at times. I called the doctor, who referred my father to the ER. A CAT scan was ordered to determine what might be causing these issues. May I say here, if your loved one has one of these procedures:

Please demand to go with them.

I started this habit with Mom, mainly because the first time she went, she was grasping my hand as if she were a child dangling off a cliff. So they agreed I could accompany her, not into the room but up the elevator and through a series of hallways where they left her in the hallway outside radiology. If I had not been there, she would have waited alone in that hallway.

Can you imagine? A dementia patient, already frightened and unable to understand what is going on, left alone on a gurney, staring at the bright, stark lights of a hospital ceiling as medical staff flurry by? I cannot. So this has become my routine. This is what I did when my daughter had a mysterious lump on the side of her neck which required a scan and it has been my routine with her much larger grandparents as well.

They completed Dad's scan and we went back to the ER to wait for the results. The doctor delivered the news. He wanted to talk to me at the nurses' station. I saw the scan clipped onto the light board behind the desk. The doctor flipped on the light. Suddenly, my knees went weak. I fell back and drifted, lifeless, onto the bench behind me. "Mrs. Ingalsbe? I need to show you something." I wept. Whatever he had to say, I could not- oh, please, not again!

"Mrs. Ingalsbe?" I opened my mouth to respond and took in a giant mouthful of salty water. I was drowning. Looking up through tears of desperation I heard him say, "We did not find anything that would explain your father's dizzy spells." I crashed into a jagged rock and held on for dear life, gasping for air. The doctor looked at me with curious sympathy. "I am just so tired," I whispered. "My brother is dead. It's just me."

"I am so sorry," he said. I climbed higher onto the rock. I would not tell him my brother had been gone for almost twenty years. "Mrs. Ingalsbe, what I need to tell you is this." He took a metal pen out of his pocket, and with a violent casting motion, transformed it into a stick, which swiftly landed on the scan.

Your father has a fairly large aneurysm here on the main artery of his heart.

He struck the sword into the scan on the precise location, as if that mattered, then violently stabbed it again into my father's heart. Blood poured out all over my soul, splashing waves of bloody water around me. A giant red wave struck as its unrelenting current knocked me off the jagged rock and pulled me under into the dangerous waters of despair. My father rested peacefully, unaware of the pain inflicted on us, unable to experience the grief.

In the days to come, more changes would be experienced, more challenges confronted. My father would be facing a move. It was imperative he have my assistance. This incredible change would be impossible for him to navigate

233

without my help. He was now totally dependent on me, and had been for some time. I would need help as well, to find the strength in which to face the realities of the future. I found myself paralyzed, literally unable to move. I was facing yet another one of the toughest decisions I have ever made.

I asked my youngest daughter, recently graduated from college, if she would find a job in our city and move home for the summer to hold my hand through this process. She agreed. Remembering how painfully difficult the move just over a decade ago was, I found myself unable to get up and take the next step. If it had not been for my daughter's hand reaching out in support, I honestly do not think I could have walked through the threshold of a single memory care facility.

Suddenly, I understood how my father felt that day at the mall. Now I was that mule, digging in my heels, adamantly rejecting any further attempts to be moved another inch. In desperation, I absolutely refused to enter. After all, this was his home, the apartment where he had carried my mother over the threshold just ten short years ago. How could I move him out of a place so familiar and into one of "those places"?

My father does not belong there!

Over a decade after his diagnosis, I was still struggling mightily accepting the fact my father was ill, his brain diseased. No longer could he manage in the apartment he had chosen long ago. Not only was he unable to manage alone, I had rallied all the troops I could afford to help him. Round-the-clock care had been in place for years. Now a team of six capable, caring women poured out their love and offered their hands of support to my father. It was not enough.

I knew there were many times one person was not sufficient strength to help my father. Often Tammy asked a friend, who assisted the centenarian neighbor across the hall, to help her. The strength required was occurring more frequently and I knew the day was coming when this would be a more than a common occurrence. My grieving heart knew nothing could guard us from facing the realities of the future. My dad needed me!

It was time to jump back in the water and face this raging storm. Securely fastening Dad's life vest, we plunged headfirst into the current. I did not know how Dad would respond to this disruption of his life. Although I was terrified at the thought of moving him, this change was inevitable. My daughter loaded me in her car before I had a chance to change my mind. By that evening, we had toured some beautiful facilities and I signed a contract for Dad's new home.

Tammy helped me sort through the belongings in Dad's apartment and carefully choose what we would pack to accompany my father to his new room at Memory Care. I carefully orchestrated a plan for Tammy to sneak him over as furniture was swiftly placed in his new room. Maybe he would not notice? Unfortunately, the movers arrived early and started carrying furniture out right in front of Dad before I could stop them. Incredibly, it did not faze him.

Dad was not physically sitting in his chair when the movers loaded it on the moving van, but I'm convinced he could have been. Isn't that a beautiful illustration of this journey we are on? It is planned out for us; the script written long ago. If we will trust, learn to slow down and ask for help by seeking wisdom and direction. If we can stop trying to control this uncontrollable disease, God will carry us! I packed Dad's bags as we boldly took this next painfully difficult step.

This is the beautiful truth: If none of this had happened, this book would not be in your possession now. Ever. It took Dad and me finding the strength to lift our feet, as well as the faith needed to place them on the next step. If we had refused, I would have never met the people, heard the stories, gained the insight, and discovered the encouragement I would need to share our story with you. There was something you needed to know. Someone knew you might be in need of some encouragement.

"Because I have a name, please find the help and strength we will need to take the next step."

Jagged Rocks

Acknowledging the anger
as we attempt to understand the pain.

I was driving down the very busy street which leads to my father's house a while ago. Traffic was even heavier than normal, I was running a little later than I had planned and hit the rush hour crowd. Soon I realized traffic was being diverted out of the lane I was in and into another. I flipped on my turn signal to get into the other lane. I was not sure where this was going, or why it was necessary. Regardless, I got the message loud and clear.

Then I saw her, standing in the middle of this very busy street, waving her arms in urgency. She obviously had a very important message.

"Go! You must move! These folks are hurt!"

I flipped my signal off and stayed in the lane I was in, having always been somewhat of a rebel anyway. There, in the middle of this city street was the Memory Care nursing director standing next to a wrecked car. I rolled down my window and called out to her:

"Are you okay? Do you need help?"

She smiled, still waving her arms and spreading her message. This representative nodded her head as she continued her work.

"Help is on the way!"

Come to find out, she was not involved in the wreck at all, she just happened on some folks that needed help. The young woman in one of the cars had three very young children. I never even saw her, she and her children were simply faceless victims of this unfortunate incident. In fact, I never saw the other driver either and I do not know if there were passengers in that car. Make no mistake about it, I saw our nursing director and I heard her message, loud and clear. Immediately, my heart filled with compassion for the young woman and her children because I heard their story.

I arrived to Memory Care, which was just a few hundred yards away. Immediately, I noticed our new director of marketing with some obviously imperative papers in her hand. She stopped at the front desk asking our receptionist where the director of nursing was "I cannot find her anywhere," she reported with frustration. "Oh, she's out there, in the middle of the street." I said, motioning and pointing, should there be any question of the street in question.

This woman who did not yet know me well scrunched her eyes and looked directly at me as if she was sizing me up. Could I be trusted? "Why would she be in the middle of the street?" she challenged. "There has been a terrible accident," I said. "Those folks need help. She is directing traffic." A look of sincere surprise was flashed my way. She paused, then said: "Well, I guess they need her help more than we do right now!" It begs to question what difference we could make if only we began to wave our arms of distress in **their** defense.

When you think about it, confusion and frustration is usually the result of not knowing what is coming next. We are in traffic, it is rerouted. We can only see so far in the horizon- the path is barely visible beyond the next turn. So we keep our eyes focused on the cars ahead of us, as we follow their lead. If we are fortunate, someone took the time to provide some much needed help. Every so often, arms are waving, warning of danger and guiding the way.

We have become a family up at Memory Care, a close knit group who looks out for one another's loved ones. We exchange hugs and knowing looks of support in the dining room. Unfortunately, it is not like PTA where we have the privilege of building years of friendships. Our lives are in constant change where saying goodbye is a common occurrence. Although I know DeAnn cannot have chocolate and Jane does not like peas, I am sorry to say I only know most family members by their first names.

We snap photos of one another's mothers and fathers and text them to each other. I receive texts and photos at least weekly from other family members, as well as the staff. I get a quick glimpse of my daddy's day, a comical moment, or something he said. My day is made! We do not want anyone to miss out on any important happening. These days are unspeakably numbered.

I took a photo of Patty and Jane the other day. They were holding hands, apparently exchanging tender words of support. Jane was patting Patty's hand; Patty offered a comforting pat in return. It was absolutely heartwarming. I was transfixed on this moment as Dad's next bite dangled from the fork in my hand. Their daughters must see this, I thought.

The residents are tight knit as well. Ann urgently stopped me yesterday as I was on my way out. "We need help over here," she said. I turned and asked how I could help. She motioned towards Cartha, who was holding her hamburger bun in the air. "I believe she wants some ketchup," she said. Cartha nodded in agreement. I am still wrapping my mind around how she knew. Would Ann have known I like mayo, not mustard, and never ketchup?

One day an aide went into my father's room to get him for lunch. Dad was gone, his chair empty and down. Apparently, at least a couple months ago, my father could still stand up on his own- on a good day. Just like you or I might do, he decided to visit his neighbor across the way. Dad was found sitting on Rex's sofa watching television with his friend.

Since you-know-who took the television out of my father's room, this seems like a reasonable proposition, right? Both men were completely content, seems they had it all worked out on their own. Dad must have extended an invitation that day because Rex has since been found sitting in Dad's guest chair exchanging pleasantries, or perhaps discussing who might have stolen Dad's television.

The staff has become like family to us as well. When our director resigned a little over a month ago, family members filed in her office to sit at her table and cry. I refused. "You will not see me cry about this," I said. She didn't. I hid in a dark corner in the privacy of my own home. God has big plans for her; I know He does. She has a huge heart and a wealth of information and insight from her decades of experience with dementia patients. I have included her website under resources at the end of the book.

Approximately two months ago I received a call in the middle of the night. From experience, I have learned it is never good news on the other end. The call alerting us to my brother's murder came in the middle of the night, as did the call I received from Aunt June to inform me of my uncle's passing. On more than one occasion I was called to the hospital in the night to be by my mother's side. One very memorable phone call alerted me of the intruder who was found wandering the halls of Assisted Living. "Your mother will have to be supervised better. Please come visit with us about this in the morning."

Each and every call from Memory Care I have received has begun with, "Your father is fine, we just wanted to let you know..." I appreciate this comforting greeting so much. Sometimes the call is about an upcoming event, Dad's blood pressure readings, or a haircut appointment. Never has a call come in the middle of the night since he has moved here. Caller ID announced the source of a 2:00am call. "Judy, this is Memory Care. First of all, I want you to know your father is fine."

Clearly he wasn't. I did not know them to make courtesy welfare announcements in the middle of the night. Dad had fallen out of the bed. He was found on the floor during a bed check. Miraculously, we (Tammy) never found a bruise on him. However, we could not afford to take any chances. We were going to need help. Hospice arrived that afternoon with a thick mat for the floor, to brace Dad's fall should he roll, or slide as the case most likely had been, out of bed again.

I continue to be astounded at the assistance and support Hospice provides us. Had I mentioned one of the directors of Hospice was instrumental in getting me to the publisher who heard my story and got this book in your hands? You will hear about it eventually. Many of the residents at Memory Care are on Hospice now. After all, this is a terminal disease. We have known this all along but it does not make the process any easier when the train turns the bend and begins its final leg of the journey into the station.

Even so, their home at Memory Care is not filled with wailing and misery as one might expect. The majority of the time, it is peaceful, even happy. One beautiful resident is fondly referred to as the centenarian, and rightfully so. Her hundred plus years of living have earned her this rare and wonderful title. Not unlike my Aunt Lennie, I suspect Mrs. B reached this milestone, in part, due to her extraordinary kindness and agreeable disposition. If cold, she kindly asks the staff to retrieve a sweater from her closet. "If it is not too much trouble," she will say.

She refuses to eat without paying for the meal. Occasionally an aide will assure her they have bought her meal for her. "Well, you are very kind." I've heard her say on more than one occasion. Other times it is a bit trickier. The other day a ticket had to be made out for her meal and delivered to her table. When Mrs. B's appetite prevents her meal from being finished, she assures staff, "It was delicious, I simply won't be able to finish." Once I heard her beseech an aide to ask "the chef" for his pumpkin pie recipe. Seems she wanted to go back to her house and make it for her family. Her thank you's are plentiful and complaints are seldom.

There are few things Mrs. B will make a fuss about, with the exception of going home. At lunch, a resident might casually mention the name of our city and the thought is rekindled. "Is that where we are?" Mrs. B asks in disbelief, "But that's so far from home!" When this desire is at its strongest, one can see this dear woman creeping her tiny walker up and down the halls. We all must keep up with the storyline, which is apparent by simply listening to the script. There are all sorts of emergencies demanding this journey be taken and all kinds of scenarios in which they take place.

Last week, Mrs. B was in her hometown and her daughter was visiting from our city. This was because her mother had fallen very ill. (Yes, the centenarian's mother, are you with me?) Dr. Williams could not come to the house and tend to her mother, as he usually did because he was in another large city in their state. I understood perfectly and offered to call Dr. Williams myself.

The desire to go home usually has little to do with home as we understand it. Some will talk incessantly about going home while residing in a house they have lived in twenty years or more. Others beg to live with their children, only to be even more unsettled once their wish is granted. We must understand the home sought no longer exists. What is longed for is a place of long ago, conjured up from memories of the past.

It may be the feeling of security and safety this memory affords them or a beloved parent they are longing for in their heart. Whatever the case, if they were taken back home, they most certainly would still be asking to go home. Too often feelings of guilt compel family members to move loved ones, or conversely, stop visiting altogether because the inability to fulfill their request is too heartbreaking.

After my mother died, although he never mentioned her by name, Dad occasionally called, "Sweetheart?" throughout the apartment. Sometimes, when coming back from a meal, he would open the door to the apartment and ask, "Is anyone here?" Tammy was quizzed more than once about "the beautiful woman that used to sit there" as he motioned towards Mom's chair.

More times than I wish to recall, Dad took a specific childhood photograph of his family off the wall and announced he was going home. Dad's drive to leave was most often due to a pressing trip to Heaven to visit his mother. Tammy's usual response was, "Yes, but we are not going today." On other occasions, Dad was simply going to the dealership to meet a gentleman who wanted to buy a car. The greatest gift we can give our loved one

247

is the feeling of safety and comfort in their home of today.

Our loved ones have lost the tools which they have had access to all their lives. They feel the emotion, sense the danger, experience the pain, but when they reach for the means to relate their feelings, the tool has mysteriously disappeared. So they turn to the abilities they have left. Maybe their two feet can take them home where they can find comfort and get some help. Perhaps they are still able to pierce their lips and shoot saliva out of their mouth, or miraculously remember a few select words from their past, which incidentally sent them to the principal's office all those years ago.

Likewise, we must reassess what is truly important. Does it really matter if mom wears mismatched clothing or if dad wants to eat his dessert before dinner? They continue to possess a will and preferences, no matter how odd they seem to us. The best gauge is to honor their choices, if they aren't harmful. This is still their life to live and if we allow them opportunity, we may find they are capable of negotiating some things quite well.
Regardless of the reality you believe to be true, they are now right- and that makes you wrong by default.

Often, we are so eager to make sense of things for our loved ones, we make it our crusade to correct every inaccurate detail of their lives. There is no need to remind dad that it was bacon, not sausage, he had for breakfast. Neither is it beneficial to correct Mom by letting her know her hair appointment was yesterday, not last week. By correcting our loved ones, we are only adding stress and agitation to their day. Before attempting to change a loved one's behavior, ask yourself these three questions:

Is what they are doing right now harming me?

Is what they are doing right now harming anyone else?

Is what they are doing right now harming them?

Their behavior may be irritating you, but this is beside the point. These guidelines can be applied to any person with dementia, this includes one who might wander into your loved one's room or be found carrying around their belongings. We must understand they are doing the best they can with the abilities they have left. Our battles have to be chosen wisely, as we learn to address only those which are disruptive.

A dementia patient's anxiety can be expressed in a variety of ways, including irritability, frustration, restlessness, demands for attention, repetitive questions, stubborn refusals, yelling, screaming, cursing, threats, hitting, kicking, biting, or spitting, just to name a few. Anxiety is most often caused by not knowing what is going to happen next. Apply this definition to your own life and see if this rings true.

I was sorting through memories with my dad today when I heard. Tom died. It hit me like a rock, crashing through my soul. Tom was a brilliant man, with a successful construction company, who was responsible for much of the architecture which graces our city's skyline. As fate would have it, the day I learned of his death was also the day a photographer was coming to take pictures for this book.

I have attempted, from the beginning, to understand why I am writing in this manner, out of order. This resembles many unanswered questions I have about this disease, Tom being one of them. A few months after my dad was settled in, Tom became a resident of this community. We were all excited for the prospect of another man joining the family. Dad's neighbor, a man with similar interests, had recently died.

Family members began the process of getting to know Tom as staff set about discovering how to make his life better. Medications were reviewed and a treatment plan was created. He had much to overcome and his behavioral issues did not make it an easy process. Tom was constantly on the move and attempting to leave the building, which begged the question, "Why?"

The mystery was not difficult to uncover. Here was a man who worked outside all of his life, overseeing the building of large buildings. It's no wonder he was not comfortable remaining indoors all day. To make matters worse, there was a building going up right beside Memory Care, the crane visible from the front windows. Tom often watched out the windows of the activity room, frustrated and unable to get the construction crew's attention to alert them of mistakes being made.

Staff thoughtfully walked Tom outside when he went to the door in an attempt to "escape." Perhaps he wasn't trying to breakout at all, but rather just get a little piece of his life back. Because of his decades of experience, he obviously had some ideas of his own about the construction process. So Memory Care staff began to ask his opinion. Tom was given a briefcase and asked to attend meetings. A world was created for him in which he could flourish, although in reality, we were all just actors in a play.

Staff was in a meeting one morning when Tom appeared at the door. The head of nursing informed him that he was ten minutes late. Tom shot her a scolding look as if to say, "How dare you talk to me that way!" "I'm the boss!" Realizing she had stepped over the line, she said, "Forgive me, sir!" Tom looked at her and said, "You're forgiven." The meeting resumed as if the incident had never happened. When Tom stepped out of the room, staff had a celebratory laugh, thankful he hadn't fired anyone. Tom flourished in this imaginary world created for him on a daily basis, most of the time.

There were contracts for Tom to sign, decisions to be made about loads of lumber or sheetrock to be ordered. They even asked his opinion on whether the guard shack should be moved to the other side of the property. Slowly, his agitation decreased and he became more pleasant, most of the time. Building projects were created for him indoors in an attempt to replace his frustration with self-worth. Following design plans, Tom built miniature picnic tables and other objects with small pieces of wood. Some days he was quite content with his newfound career, other days he clearly was not.

I arrived towards the end of lunch to visit Dad a couple of months ago; the dining room was full. I found my father at a table of men, Tom standing over them, obviously upset. He had some files and was mumbling about something which apparently had gone terribly wrong. My father, obviously shaken, looked from the files, to Tom, then back. Only my father knows what was going through his mind at that moment. Perhaps he was in a meeting being reprimanded for a job poorly done, or a disgruntled employee was angry for being fired. What I do know is this: my dad had not eaten a bite of lunch.

Tom believed he owned the entire building. He was welcomed into the offices, anytime, where he looked over plans and advised the staff which wall to move or what needed to be added. He was simply carrying out his job. Rex watched, wide-eyed, as Tom stood over the men, shuffling through paperwork and angrily motioning. Dad was visibly scared. The aides, who had been busy feeding Jane, Ural, and DeAnn, residents totally dependent on their care, quickly redirected Tom to another room. It was time for him to get back to work, perhaps he had a board meeting to attend. He seemed to be drawn to the men residents and I am quite certain it angered him to find them sleeping on the job.

One day, Tom approached me in the hallway to review a project which was being done. He found me sitting at the table discussing my father's condition with Hospice. My usual tactic of smiling and mirroring everything in a positive light was not always effective with Tom. For whatever reason, my smiles seemed to disgust him. He often mocked me as my attempts to enter his world fell terribly short. I was a trigger. Perhaps I reminded him of an unqualified woman who once worked for him, or maybe he found me irritatingly friendly. Whatever the case, make no mistake, Tom did not like me.

He spotted me at the table signing the papers which would place my father on Hospice care, our daughter beside me for moral support. Putting my own set of problems aside for a moment, I turned to greet Tom as he raged towards me. Obviously there was, once again, a mistake made. Clearly, I was to blame. The innocent members of my table watched as Tom relayed the details of this particular project to me. "That's wonderful news, Tom," I said. "No, it's not!" he defiantly shouted.

The independent caregiver who was walking with him attempted to redirect, but his reprimand was not complete. I had apparently wreaked havoc on this project and there was a price to pay. When I determined there would be no resolution reached, not knowing what else to do, I simply turned around in my chair. I attempted to resume a meeting of my own, which was also of great importance. This enraged Tom and he began to thrash his walker into the back of my chair, angrily reciting my transgressions. Everyone at the table was stunned. What could we do? I thought about my father across the hall, growing more vulnerable every day. If Tom were this violent towards him, he would certainly hurt him.

Tom often went into other resident's rooms. When he relentlessly attempted to get into locked areas of the complex, a caution tape with an "out of order" sign redirected him without anyone speaking a word. This worked, for the most part, but there was only so much tape on the roll and Tom was a very busy man. He often went into my father's room, rearranging his pictures, rifling through his bathroom cabinets, stealing his glasses. The day Tammy relayed she had arrived to find Dad's guest chair leg broken and picture frames strewn about, the telltale sign of Tom's handiwork, I had heard enough.

Tom had recently slapped Rex in the dining room for no apparent reason, aggressively cussed out my daddy as he sat motionless and scared, even broke Patty's wheelchair. We all had high hopes when Tom returned from a stint in a diagnostic center that things would be different. These facilities provide psychiatric treatment and specialized medication analysis to stabilize patients in an attempt to get behaviors under control. This is the facility my mother was admitted to when she was diagnosed.

Interestingly, Tom had the same doctor who treated my mom. She was also the doctor who was able to get my father's aggressive behaviors under control in the early stages of his disease. I do not pretend to know what Tom's family was going through, nor can I fathom the extent of energy, effort, and research Memory Care poured into a care plan for this man. I will never understand Tom's torment and anguish. What I do know is this: our system gave up on this man and failed to recognize him as a human being, -one in desperate need of help.

The same system, which came in for a routine check and determined Tammy could no longer so much as touch my father, much less give him a shower, discharged Tom that day. Despite their best efforts, Memory Care could not persuade the health department to allow Tom to stay and he was sent away. In the following month he was moved multiple times and quickly succumbed to the stress of it all. Consequently, our director left, too, feeling immensely defeated and discouraged for being so impossibly unable to save this man.

I do not want to give the glowing impression I was on the front lines, waving the green flag for Tom. There were times I was so frustrated and fearful for my dad's safety, as well as other residents, I would have opened the front door myself. If I am honest, there have been moments in my own journey I just wanted to lock the door and shield myself from my own parents' issues. There will be these points in all of our journeys in which we are beat down from the waves relentlessly crashing on us, violently slamming us into the next jagged rock, that we want to give up on it all. We will want to give up on them.

There will be times we are so cut from the pain and bloody from the heartbreak we will want to quit. Drag ourselves up onto the shore and just walk away. We are strong enough, you know, even in our weakened, battered state. We have taken in mouthfuls of salty water, you and I, which left us gasping for air. You know we have enough in us to swim to safety. We are capable, able to plot a course of escape and make it out of these uncompromising currents. However, we dare not think this way. You and I both know we cannot take *them* with us.

We must cling to the next jagged rock we find, hanging onto our loved ones for dear life, pulling them above water. You and I are going to have to ride out this storm. At times we will need to take out our distress signal and call for help. There will be seasons of such excruciating pain we will need to get reinforcements to help so we can throw ourselves onto the rock and recover. Then we must get back in the water. *They* are counting on it. There have been too many casualties already.

Tom is just one story of a life which once held so much significance, a man who was such an incredible asset to our community. He found himself on a jagged rock which wounded anyone who dared to get close, even those who were just trying to find something to hold onto in order to survive the next current themselves. We failed him. All of us. This disease demands our attention. We need answers we simply do not have and we need them quickly. It is time we call in reinforcements, ask our legislators for help, and get our loved ones fitted with life vests. This storm will not calm until we do.

"Because I have a name, please do not give up on me."

Staying Afloat

*Grabbing a life vest for our loved ones
as we jump in the water right along with them.*

One of the sweet ladies at Memory Care had not
experienced the glorious pleasure of a bath or a shower
in over a year when she moved in. Can you imagine?
She lived alone. Her family brought in meals, did
laundry, and kept her house clean. They did everything
they could to keep her going in her home for as long as
they could. Eventually, they realized there were never
any towels in the wash, only washcloths. When asked if
she was bathing, she assured them she was. It became
terribly apparent she was not.

These folks do not want to jump in these waters any
more than we do, and these are the stories I just happen
to have heard about. One of the men downright threw a
fit the other day and sent the Hospice nurse packing.
She emerged from the raging waters to announce, "I will
be back tomorrow to try again." After raging out of the
shower covered in soap and shampoo, a sedative
beforehand will be tried to see if he might be a bit more
agreeable to the necessary process.

So although it seems obvious tips would be helpful, that perhaps your loved one has the same issues, that is not exactly what this chapter is about. Instead, it is the tale of this one, explaining to you how I have managed to keep my head above water. Many, many times I have felt like I was drowning in this disease. Especially of late, I have found it increasingly difficult to keep my father afloat. Perhaps you feel the same way.

One day, the health department came to Memory Care for a routine check. They were there for three days, interviewing staff and families, going through records, examining routines, spreading stress like wildfire. At least that is how I perceived it. I had my hands full at the time. Seems to be a common occurrence nowadays. The previous director, my friend, even asked me if I had called in the health department. She knew I was angry, but I did not call. As far as I know, no one did. They just came, as they will every year.

In fact, when the investigator stopped by my father's room to ask if we had any problems with the place, if I had any concerns or complaints, I told her we had none. "We have some great aides here," I said, "Some amazing, caring people. We just need more like them." It just so happened three of my favorites were working that morning. "You don't think they have enough help?" she asked. That was not what I said.

I had this conversation with this investigator after she thought to ask me. She had first attempted to ask my father questions after I relayed to her the fact my father has been suffering with this disease for over a decade. You may have guessed this tactic did not work out so well for her. "Hello, sir," Dad roused up from a catnap in his enormous, oversized recliner covered in a blanket of his alma-mater's colors, hands, shaking with tremors, folded in his lap. This woman, sporting a clipboard, did not so much as step foot inside my father's room on this occasion, although I offered her the guest chair.

Her questions were posed from the other side of the threshold, as if we were some kind of freak show, some woman's place she was not willing to enter. Please hear me when I say this: I am not blaming her. We have but one enemy and we need to wage war on this disease. There is so much misinformation, too much misunderstanding, surrounding this mysterious disease, which apparently results in folks not remembering who we are. The Health Department was simply doing their job, trying to keep our loved ones safe. For this, I am grateful.

"Hello," Dad states, staring blankly at her. He blinks. She continues to look over her clipboard, as she prepares to collect pertinent information for her report. "Sir, could you tell me how long you have been here?" She is met with a blank stare. I wanted to tell her she would not be able to interview my dad in this way, that he would not respond to questions such as these. I was wrong. "A hundred years," he stated. Come to find out, he was able to answer.

She directed the next question to me. "What about his care? Do you feel like they are keeping him clean?" That struck a nerve. This is what I was so angry about. My father had been gotten out of bed before Tammy arrived, dressed, and taken to the dining room for breakfast before he had a shower. Tammy is the one who comes each morning to shower him, to ensure he is clean each day. Everyone knows this. I have made sure of that. If this were not in place, I do not know what we would do.

The staff is busy getting all the residents up, toileted, dressed, and taken to the dining room in the mornings. They then serve them breakfast. On any given morning there are at least three who are totally dependent on the aides to get food to their mouths. Daddy makes four increasingly frequently. Can you imagine what an undertaking this is? Not to mention someone is on the med cart doling out necessary medications every resident requires, all with their own set of specific instructions how they are to be taken. Additionally, my father's medicine has to be crushed now, he will not take them otherwise.

This process started almost a year ago. We had to drop the vitamins because they are simply too large and there are approximately six medications, treating the Alzheimer's, Parkinson's, depression, and anxiety that are pertinent to his well-being. Gone are the days he threw them all in his mouth and swallowed in one swift gulp. So they are crushed and put in applesauce or yogurt. One of the aides (because Tammy is not allowed to) painstakingly feeds him every bite. I do not know how many other residents require such a process. Tammy could tell you. She is there for breakfast five days a week.

So this is why we have this arrangement in place, for Tammy to come each morning. This gets Dad's day off to the best possible start to see my "sister's" smiling face and experience their predictable routine. Once Dad wakes, Tammy begins the process of getting him out of bed. This sometimes requires the help of one or two of the aides, at other times Tammy and Dad work together and are able to manage on their own. They have been a team for a long time now and understand the personality and specific idiosyncrasies of one another.

I became keenly aware of this the day, approximately five years ago, when I received a call from Tammy to report happenings of their walk along the little trail which went around the small pond on the property. This pond was visible from the window of Dad's apartment. I suspect he viewed it each morning as the caregivers drew his blinds to entice a greeting of the day. Perhaps the pond offered fond memories of the "lake", as he proudly called it, at his beloved apartment complex.

Tammy called to report my father had relieved himself by a tree on their little excursion, "Right there outside the dining room." I was horrified! "I tried my best to stop him," she continued, "but when he has to go, he's got to go!" We tried our best to be on our best behavior there. After all, this was independent living and these folks did not want to live with individuals who "belonged in the nursing home."

In fact, when my mother came back from one of her stints in the hospital and required the help of her caregivers in order to eat, she was banned from the dining room. They did not care that she had temporarily lost the use of her hand from a stroke she suffered. They just wanted her out. I told the powers that be my parents would eat in their apartment until she was better. The director offered us the card room, separate from the other folks. We accepted. It was a change of scenery for my parents and afforded them some exercise, as well as similar routine. So we hid our nasty little problem in there.

I would deal with this as well, should someone have happened to witness my father hesitating on his walk. This issue had been going on for some time, relieving himself in unusual places throughout the apartment. It is a common occurrence with these folks and happens fairly early on in the disease process. Now, after over a decade, there is absolutely no control at all, for any bodily function. Most of the time, Tammy arrives to find him covered: soaked and dirty.

This is why she comes faithfully, it is why I have signs throughout his bathroom and in his closet. *"Please! Do not dress Bob before he has a shower!"* Should an aide find him in this condition during a routine check before Tammy arrives, they (should) know to take him straight to the shower. I am quite certain my father is familiar with such rules. After sitting in the dirt all day with his boy scout buddies, tirelessly building sets of wings for future experiments, I can picture him running through the door of his childhood home. Just in time for dinner he would race in, only to hear his mother say: *"Straight to the shower, young man!"*

The incident in question had occurred just a few short days before this particular day, which brought this woman to the threshold of my father's home questioning his life and threatening his future. Tammy arrived to find my father, covered in the functions of the night before, dressed, sitting in the dining room eating the only way he knew, sans prompting, with his hands. She was furious. I was enraged. This was the second time this had happened, and believe me when I say, folks heard about this.

I cannot speak for everyone, but I would venture to say most of us have thoroughly considered bringing our loved ones' home to care for them ourselves. I know my husband and I have. Something like this occurs and we think, we can do a better job of this ourselves. However, we know in our hearts we cannot. I should say, since I can only speak for myself-I cannot. My father requires too much assistance now and it takes a team to accomplish this. We all must work together for his benefit. That means we are going to have to get along, even on the worst days when someone makes a mistake.

If the truth be known, there are many loving, caring individuals who pour out their hearts, reading the scripts of their patient's realities, as they write them meal tickets and dance these folks to the bathroom. These aides have become like family to me, too. We sit at mealtime together as we enter each other's lives. They come to my father's room and borrow the residents' favorite music CD's to listen to in the common's room. Hoisting my father to his feet, they encourage him to dance, and send me pictures.

I walked in the other day to a wonderful song which lifted my spirits and warmed my heart. As I turned the corner I saw one of my favorites coming toward me. Instantaneously, we both turned to the side, skipping and dancing as we passed in the hall. I have met their children, heard their stories, and attempted to become a part of their lives- in all the spare moments we have when not meeting my father's needs.

When I discovered who had taken Dad to the dining room in this condition, I was devastated. She was one of my favorites as well. (Who am I kidding? I love them all.)

They sacrifice for my father every, single day. I had asked the director about this particular favorite just weeks before, mentioning I had not seen her in a long time and hoped she had not left. She went home for the holidays and would be returning soon, the director assured me.

I spotted her coming through the door a few days later and we greeted each other with a giant hug. There are no ill feelings towards her for what she did. I hope these words make it to her someday. I am not upset with her. She made a mistake. Lord knows I have too, and I do not bear even a portion of the burden these aides do in caring for my father. I am not angry with her, but I will continue to pick up my father's wet towel off the floor and wave it in the air, demanding his dignity and insuring his well-being.

I have not seen this aide in quite a while. I fear she was dismissed. The first aide to have done this was escorted off the property by the police. Perhaps she was just moved to the other building. I may never know, unless I get up the courage to ask. To every single one of you who provide care for my father and the other forty-four million victims of Alzheimer's disease worldwide; I know you do not hear this often enough:

Thank you.
You are appreciated and valued,
more than you will ever know!

A few days after the health department paid a visit, I was called into the director's office. The news she and the owner, down from another state to help carry out the orders, were delivering was worse than I could have ever imagined. Tammy would no longer be allowed to shower my father. Additionally, she would not be able to so much as touch him to provide care of any kind-to take him to the restroom, brush his teeth, tie his shoe. I was devastated.

"Can I give him a shower?" I asked. They explained that I could because I am family, although it came with a warning. "Judy, you don't want to do that. It would make your father terribly uncomfortable. The aides can give him a shower." I knew they already had more than enough to do and I am the first to admit, providing a shower each morning at a specific time is a monumental request. "But Tammy is my sister," I pleaded. "She has facilitated his showers for almost ten years!" "I know you think of her as a sister," the director consoled, "but they are not going to allow her to come in anymore."

The same wave which swept Tammy out into the current, taking my father with her, had swept Tom out to sea as well. The health department determined he was a risk to the other residents and sent him packing. The director even offered to move him to an empty building, not yet filled with a single resident, and provide aides to care for him over there. That was not good enough. My father used to say he believed folks often placed rules over common sense. I believe this was such an example.

Ultimately, Memory Care sent out a search and rescue squad for me. They retrieved Tammy and my father from the choppy waters, offering to hire her for the sole purpose of facilitating Dad's showers in the morning. This was the issue the state had: Memory Care was not her employer-I was. I am grateful beyond words they were willing to do this for me-for my father. The director and corporate jumped many hurdles, navigating numerous threatening waves to make this happen.

Thank you. I am so very grateful.

My father may not know exactly how long he has lived at Memory Care, nor be capable of getting out of bed by himself any longer. He has not spoken my name in years and may not even have a recollection of my face some days. For whatever reason, I am becoming increasingly invisible to him of late. He simply does not see or hear me at all and that is one I did not see coming. My father struggles mightily to make it through each day.

However, when he hears the water running in the bathroom and Tammy's voice singing as she turns on the music, "Good morning, Mr. Bob!" When he walks the familiar steps as she leads him to the toilet. Then picks up his leg and steps way over the side of the tub, although there has not been such a tub to step over since he moved out of his apartment almost nine months ago. When Tammy helps him sit down on the shower chair and begins to wash his hands and painstakingly clean under his fingernails.

When she gently washes his hair as she hands him a washcloth and asks him to wipe his eyes, then guides his hand to clean inside his ears. He knows exactly what to do. When she hands him his toothbrush, reminding him how to put it in his mouth and move it up and down and round and round on his teeth, he routinely follows the practice they have been perfecting for many years. She then shaves my father, explaining what she is doing as she goes, the same process she has carried out every day for all these years.

Before he is wrapped in a warm towel, his body is washed. He is now ready for a good day. He has been provided the best possible beginning to ensure the most marvelous day imaginable. He will continue to have good days and bad days, but this gift is acknowledged. It is not that no one else could do this. The aides at Memory Care who showered him while Tammy was sent out to sea, and continue to keep him clean on Sundays while she is enjoying a rare day off, do a great job, as does the Hospice aide who comes on Wednesdays.

The fact is, my father and Tammy have a dance, a well-practiced production they have now perfected. When Dad picks up his foot and takes that first step, suddenly he knows the dance and he simply moves to the beat.

They are swept here and there in the crashing waves far too often, slammed against rocks and washed up to shore, breathless. They need to know what to expect and that does not happen by running in the room saying, "Time for a shower!" as their clothes are snatched off by strangers.

They need a dance.
Please find one they enjoy and begin the practice today.

Too often we get caught up on the wrong issues, like if our loved one remembers us. Folks ask me this question all the time. Sadly, it is tempting to measure our worth on the answer. In social settings, a family member may share their loved one's condition and inevitably, the concerned listener will ask, "Do they still know who you are?" Although well meaning, this question is not relevant and potentially hurtful.

The question suggests that whether the individual can recall a name or recognize a face is a determining factor of the quality of the relationship. This inquiry has been made of me numerous times over the years and, quite frankly, I do not know whether my dad has an understanding that I am his daughter or not. For all you who are curious: It no longer matters if I am recognized and I am not saddened by the proposition.

The question used to frighten me. "What if he doesn't know who I am?" I could think of nothing more heartbreaking than to be caring for and loving a person who did not have the slightest idea who I was. Surely if I visited more often or was doing an exceptional job of caring for my parents they would recognize me. The fact is, much of the time, dementia patients do not even recognize themselves in the mirror.

I have learned to embrace the irony of the disease and laugh at the humor it sometimes affords. One Christmas, early on in the disease process when I would have guaranteed that my parents knew who I was, this story was relayed to me. A caregiver was with my parents when one of their dear friends called. She had received a Christmas card from my parents, which I had sent. Hoping to generate welcomed greetings from friends and family, I was in the habit of sending cards out on my parents' behalf.

Dad answered the phone and his friend, who he struggled to recall, wished him a Merry Christmas. "Judy wrote a little note with your card this year," she said. "Who did?" Dad responded. "Your daughter, Judy," she replied. Dad excused himself from the phone. He turned to my mom and asked if she knew anyone named Judy. After thoughtful consideration, she assured him that she did not.

Over the years I have become much less concerned over the issue of being known. I know my parents and this is all that matters to me. The mystery of what my dad knows or does not know is irrelevant in comparison to the indescribable connection I feel with him. I no longer ask if

275

he knows my name, but instead pose the question, "Do you know how much I love you, Dad?" Thankfully, the measure of my relationship with my dad is not dependent on his capacity to remember me.

I always give my dad a kiss on the cheek when I greet him. Sometimes his eyes will pop open and he will say, "Wowie!!" At other times a slight smile comes over his face. Whatever his reaction, I know that he experiences my love. If I want to really make him happy, I scratch his back. He loves to have his back and shoulders rubbed, so this is often his reward for standing up.

After doing just that recently, Dad and I were walking down the hall when a staff member struck up a conversation. He asked my father if he knew who I was, which was met with a quizzical look. Perhaps out of curiosity, but more than likely just seeking to encourage conversation, the staff member pressed on asking, "Do you know this lady's name?" as he gestured towards me. "That's no lady," my dad responded. "She's my little girl, Goofy!"

Dad has made a bit of a habit of referring to me by this name recently and I hold the title proudly. I have learned to celebrate those moments of connection when I can almost dismiss the fact anything is wrong. Years ago, when I was silly, my dad would pick up a banana and call "The Funny Farm" to come pick me up. This is perhaps the brightest glimmer of recognition I have found in this disease in many years.

We must lay aside our preconceived ideas of how things should be and begin to enjoy the realities of life as it is. I joined my dad and his buddy, Rex, recently for lunch. The magical moment arrived as cookies were served, even to those not finishing their meal. These folks have earned a cookie or two, regardless of their present performance. Rex picked up his cookie and ate a bite, which rendered it half-eaten, then returned it to his plate.

This cued my father to reach his immensely long arm across the table and swipe the remaining bite of his friend's cookie. I would say I was horrified, but this would be a lie. This behavior happens on a daily basis now and I have grown accustomed to the sharing of meals. However, I continue to occasionally need a reminder to stop correcting my father. "Dad!" I exclaimed, "That is Rex's cookie! Yours is over here!" As I stood to retrieve it out of his hand, Rex intercepted my mission.

The words he spoke were filled with wisdom, compassion, and a loyalty few possess. "It's okay!" he stated, holding his hand up in defiance. "We will work it out." Who knew they were not in need of a mediator? I failed to acknowledge the fact these two gentlemen could navigate their friendship quite well on their own. I will never forget their faces when I left that day; they were looks of complete contentment. Perhaps we could learn a thing or two about sharing cookies.

"Because I have a name, please focus less on what I can recall and simply enjoy our dance."

Fishing Off the Pier

Because He heard our cries, help is on the way!

I know now this is why I am writing this book. It is not about my family's story, nor is it about simply offering you some encouragement, although I hope and pray I have. It is about **them** and I would have done it all again for **them**. But hear me when I say if I had known, truly understood, all the difficult and impossible things God was going to call me to do, I would have been convinced I could not handle them on my own and I would have been right.

He is my lifeline; the strength I am counting on to walk with me.

It strikes me that our Father has to communicate with us in the same manner I have been suggesting you communicate with your loved one. Enter their reality, because they are not capable of entering ours. They do not possess the capability to understand.

Neither do we.

Just as this reality we live is very real to us, experienced in a tangible, meaningful way, **their** reality is real to them. We are not entering a world of pretend, we are joining **their** reality. If you think about it, we are not much different from these folks. We become anxious when we attempt to enter God's world and understand the future. When **they** are forced to enter ours, **they** become anxious as well.

Explaining details or the reasoning behind
every situation or decision is not productive.
Your role is to help; this is all any of us would be seeking.
Simply relay this beautiful fact and repeat as necessary:

I will help you; I will take care of everything.

Do you see it? This is what God is doing with us. Our brains simply do not have the capacity to understand it all. I did not even see this coming, and believe me when I say, I have tried to figure this out many times.

Here we are expending all of this effort, eager to make sense of things for our loved ones, making it our crusade to correct every inaccurate detail of their lives, when they seem to have a better grasp of reality then we do. For example, have you ever noticed they do not hold grudges? The reason is because they are not living in the past. They are not capable of going back there. Perhaps we could learn a thing or two from these folks.

I enjoyed getting to meet Joann, my friend's mother- in- law immensely. She is a beautiful, articulate woman. I told her when she left I wanted to get together for lunch again. "Well, I don't drive anymore so I will have to bring her with me," she replied as she motioned to my friend. As wonderful as the lecture series was that I attended last fall, the greatest gift I received was this friendship. I absolutely cannot imagine life absent of my friend and her family. Even the shortest of texts, usually right before we jump back into these unknown waters to work out another day, offer encouragement, strength, and a heaping dose of shared faith.

JoAnn is passionate about her faith as well. During lunch she shared her burden for those who do not acknowledge Jesus as Savior. She has invested countless hours reading their stories, trying to better understand their beliefs, and praying for them. "I just know there is more I could do." I suggested she write a letter and make numerous copies which could be mailed as those she is concerned about are brought to mind. This legacy could live on long after she is gone.

Many mornings these two beautiful ladies are brought to mind as a smile sweeps over my face. A beautiful, caring woman with a huge heart who realizes how much God has blessed her and counts on Him to give her the wisdom and patience to walk through life on a daily basis with her mother-in-law. I cannot think of a more beautiful way of thanking this woman for raising her husband. My friend writes:

> *I think sometimes it is good for other people*
> *to see how things are with our loved ones.*
> *In general, I think people might think*
> *that it's an easy thing to do.*
> *So that's why I have friends that are*
> *going through the same thing and go to events*
> *that The Alzheimer's Association puts out.*
> *They can be helpful in offering*
> *support and understanding what it's like.*
>
> *That is why I said "sometimes"*
> *because I don't want to burden or bore anyone.*

It is interesting to me; we are never bored with the stories of other family members. Conversely, they are familiar and strangely comforting. It is as if we are on a lifeboat and the sight of another lifeboat gives us hope, the knowledge we are not alone in this storm and the strength required to make it through the night.

We must look beyond the disease and delight in the individual and their unique personality. The reason for our hurry will not be remembered years from now, but the treasured moment will. Slow down and enjoy! Often just by being present in the moment, will afford our loved ones a beautiful experience. In the past few months, my dad and I have found beautiful moments reading a love story together.

The quiet, sweet, articulate girl had won over the charming, witty young man. Bob spent Sundays after church getting to know her family and enjoying her Mother's wonderful meals. Betty's brothers taught Bob to play dominoes under the old Pecan tree in the backyard. She enjoyed long drives in his car, picnicking at the lake, and discussing the future. Bob determined he couldn't live without her and transferred to OU the next semester. It wasn't long before they were dreaming dreams and making promises only commitment, determination, and love can keep.

Dad interrupted my reading for just a moment to fill me in on an important detail, "That's me!" he exclaimed. "That's right, Dad. This story is about you and your sweetheart."

When Betty June was stricken with pneumonia and they had to be apart, she visited you daily. You would notice your sweetheart coming up the corridor, and you ran as a sprinter- just like you did in track. You reached out your arms, not wanting another moment to pass without holding your sweetheart.

Dad smiled, then blinked, his eyes wide in eager anticipation of soaking in the next word.

When you reached her, you held her and told her you loved her. "Have you come to see me?" you asked. Betty June smiled and said, "You are the love of my life." It was as if you two had loved each other forever, because you had.

283

"Beautiful," Dad commented. "Yes, she was, Dad, and you were a wonderful husband." These folks are much more insightful than we give them credit for. Remember Jane? Although she rarely talks, she loves music and conversationally visited with my father during a musical one evening, which stunned us all. Deep down inside she knows who she is and she certainly still has a will. Her daughter told me her mother recently made this request of her: "Don't feed me peas."

I can relate to this request. Although I happen to love peas, as a child I would not eat chicken, and for good reason. One of the carefully chosen pictures displayed on Dad's wall is a small photo of a blonde haired girl holding an enormous white leghorn chicken. I may be a city girl, but I do know my chickens. The lovely animal in the photo was my pet, D.D., named after my elementary school. She lived in our backyard for five years, right up to the fateful night now in question.

This beloved pet would be the reason Dad spent an entire weekend of his life building an elaborate chicken coop. She would be the cause for my mom to carefully glue egg shells back together, then number them. This was done, I suppose, in case we ever became curious as to just how many eggs D.D. laid in her lifetime and were inclined to dig through boxes in the attic for absolute proof. I am quite certain this was my clever idea.

D.D.'s appearance in our lives also subsequently led to five roosters and a Rhode Island Red hen briefly residing in the backyard of our city home. The hen, Lucky, was my favorite of the brood. Smaller than her adoptive mother, she grew up to lay brown eggs-a reflection of her darker color. D.D., of course was large and white, therefore laying larger, white eggs. Isn't it interesting that life works that way? Each person, or chicken as the case may be, a unique reflection of themselves?

Their brief stint as boarders was ended when the roosters began to crow which, from my recollection, did not take long. This surrogate mother tale requires a rather elaborate explanation of how my grandma came to borrow fertile eggs from a local farmer. This is a story for another day. The point is, none of these things would have occurred had I not triumphantly won the drawing. The prize acquired was a baby chick, hatched as a science experiment in my first grade class.

This fuzzy yellow bundle, which easily fit in my tiny hand, was soon to be christened D.D. Make no mistake, I

285

would have never been allowed to enter the drawing had my parents thought there was a chance, at any location this side of heaven, I would win. To their amazement and disdain, I did. In time, however, even they grew to love that chicken. Yes, even my dad. He truly loved our resident pet chicken. Perhaps it was the joy this beloved animal brought me that he treasured most. This is why the morning he stopped me short of the backdoor was so painfully difficult.

As was my normal morning routine, I was heading out the backdoor to feed my pet. Dad intercepted my chore and relayed the terrible news. D.D. had died of a heart attack. I was not even aware this was possible, but then I was only in fifth grade. There were many things I did not yet know. Later that day, when I returned from a tear-filled day at school, we buried my beloved pet. Dad officiated. I was devastated. We all mourned the loss fervently. All of my elementary school classmates will tell you, that chicken was special.

Several years ago, I found myself looking through a picture album with my father. "Look at this picture, Dad," I said, "there I am holding D.D.!" He gazed lovingly at the image of his daughter holding this beautiful animal. Obviously, this photo had sparked a recollection.

He smiled. "She was a good pet," I said. "Too bad that cat got her," he lamented. Horrified, I dropped the photo and directed my attention to the architect of the chicken coop. "But Dad," I pleaded, "you told me D.D. died of a heart attack!" "Well, I imagine she did," he chuckled.

> *"Because I have a name, never stop sharing stories and photographs with me!"*

Stone Benches

Reflecting on the stone benches of life
and embracing each precious moment.

My father will take one look at the front cover of this book and a million beachside memories will be at his disposal. He will look at the picture of us sitting on the bench and I guarantee something will be triggered in his memory bank. They were our memories; do you see how this works? We sit on many benches during our lifetime. They are tangible representations of the moments our journey has afforded.

A stone bench inhabiting the backyard during my daughters' childhood days was where memories were made, secrets were shared, and shoes had been tied. This memorable bench also happened to be the location of my dad's favorite Easter egg hideaway. Another bench, equally as treasured, would, in later years, provide a convenient hideaway from "women's places" at the mall.

Campfire benches, many decades earlier, hosted boy scouts as they acquired the knowledge that lids should be removed before roasting beans. Two of these mischievous boys grew up to be men who discussed business on picnic benches during lunch breaks. These gentlemen would escort their beautiful dates to dinner in their golden years, and offer a padded bench for the wait.

Both men eventually sat in doctors' offices on benches which supported the sudden faintness of unwelcome news. Ultimately, a bench is where my father would find his friend, waiting in the lobby of a retirement home, for an afternoon visit and much welcomed car ride. It struck me that empty benches had also become relevant moments in our lives.

A deserted bench, the result of my lack of supervision, had rendered me frantic and, most significantly, my mother lost. The bench I found at the airport, vacant, yet willing to wait it out with me, just outside the men's restroom. These moments reinforced how valuable my parents are to me, as did the stone bench which held my mourning body in the courtyard of the funeral home.

These are our broken pieces- the heartache we hid as we sat in our corners holding tightly to our pain. We are now boldly displaying them for all to see. Coming together. Standing strong. We each begin stacking our stories, one on top of the other, until a wall of strength and fortitude is built. They already know this. We are just catching up. They have been coming together and sharing since the moment we allowed them to be brought together. These folks count on one another, look after each other, and communicate in ways we do not begin to understand.

There is a pact I have made with myself, but on days when I realize one of our family members has died, it is really hard to keep this promise. I will not let my mind go there, to the day Dad or one of his buddies crosses over the horizon, just past where we can see and enjoy them. To the bench where Pitchford sits, telling grand and glorious tales with my granddad and Uncle Bill. I must not be selfish when my father decides it is time to join them.

Grieving is such an interesting experience when our loved one has dementia. I can think of no other circumstance where the person has changed so much, yet remains the same. It is an extended period of grieving a loved one we have lost and the capabilities they cannot retrieve. By the time Mom died, I had grieved the mother I lost years before. My tears were now for this woman I had grown to love, the one I danced with in the middle of the living room. The one who brushed my hair with her fingers. The one who did not know my name.

I have, unfortunately, bore more than what I consider to be my fair share of grief in my lifetime. None is more significant than the other, no death more tragic, no loss leaving more of a void on this earth than another. Some, however, require much more support and faith to get through. There are tragedies so raw, too difficult to explain, in which we have no choice but to collapse into the arms of our Savior and weep until we draw enough strength from Him to be hoisted to our feet and nudged along the path in front of us.

Despite all these emotions, we must learn to experience joy, by cultivating gratefulness. My dear, sweet, as Dad would say, "feisty" mom who gracefully and often comically traveled the last decade of her life holding the hand of Alzheimer's is missed every day.
Despite the void I feel, there truly is so much to be thankful for, even in the midst of this terrible disease. I am especially thankful that I am here to take care of Dad.

We are marching out of the shadows and into the light to expose this disease.

I am just one person. It is going to take all of us telling our stories. Standing up and saying, "I've had enough of this heartache!" It is going to take a willingness to let the

291

anger rage up inside of us until we cannot help but wage all-out war on our common enemy of this disease. Over forty-four million folks in the world woke up this morning trying to make sense of another day with a brain that is diseased and dying. Doesn't this make you mad?

This disease will be sorry it ever messed with my family. There were already too many suffering with its effects for it to come knocking on our door. It will regret ever so much as stepping on the front porch of our lives. I am waging war! Let the same be said of you. It is going to take all of us to fight this disease. Won't you join me?

We can do so much more than simply survive another day.

Because of this disease, we all are familiar with anger, "Why did this have to happen to our loved one?" We are also met with *their* anger which is often directed at us. So we realize this disease is our common enemy and it is okay to be mad about it. This, in turn, will, hopefully, eventually motivate us to join the efforts to support the campaign for a cure. At some point we must come out of the shadows and bring this disease into the light.

I believe the most damaging monster in our arsenal of emotions is guilt. I do not have to define this one. We all spend way too much time entertaining guilt-what we should have, could have, would have done. We must learn to offer and accept grace. We all do the very best we can to manage this disease loaded with responsibilities. Answers are needed and it is time we put our insecurities aside and ask for some help.

Although we are caring for loved ones who are very much alive, the grieving process started the day they were diagnosed. It is experienced when we reach for the phone to ask Dad's advice or get that recipe from Mom. We grieve who they were and the parent, or spouse, we have lost, the relationship we had. At the same time, we set about discovering who they have become, these changing personalities. At some point, hopefully, we stop grieving the person we have lost and begin to embrace this "new person" we have to love.

When the weather is pleasant, the doors at Memory Care are opened to a beautiful little courtyard. After joining my father for a meal recently, I turned to him after the last crumb of cookie was picked from his plate and asked hopefully, "Shall we go for a little walk?" He responded with the predictable answer, "Yes." This meant he either did or did not want to go. Time would be the ultimate indicator. The cumbersome process of propelling him to his feet commenced, requiring the assistance of myself and two aides. To my delight, Dad then followed my lead towards the open door.

The wheels of Dad's walker turned deliberately, slowly, as we made our way up the pathway. When we approached the gazebo, Dad spied a bench under its shade. "That's it," he said. "Would you like to sit down?" I asked. Obviously, he did. So we accepted the invitation of the bench. The chirping of birds and intermittent breezes reminded me just how beautiful this day was. We sat in silence, as we now often do. When Dad was ready to communicate, he would alert me with a whistle. If I was fortunate, we would enjoy a concert today. This, however, could not be forced. For now, we simply soaked in the experience of being.

It was an incredible, yet insignificant moment; one which warms the heart and delights the soul nonetheless. Time taught me just how important these moments are. We were in the presence of each other, what an incredible gift. How many times had we inhabited a bench, much like the one we were sitting on now, convenient and welcoming? They hosted the most memorable occasions of our lives. A bench, as significant as the one Dad and I were now sitting on, invited my parents to enjoy priceless promise-making moments under the Oak tree.

Through the years, those promises had been strengthened with prayers on church pews. Eventually, they were realized on hospital benches awaiting the birth of grandchildren and train station platforms as my parents traveled the world. Decades later, my father made his way to a warm stone bench to take in the serenity of the ocean and reflect on a love well lived. We now found ourselves here, in the courtyard of Dad's Memory Care. I held his hand, as well as the precious memories he could not.

What he could do, and this is of great significance, was experience the beautiful moment which now enveloped us. He could find enjoyment in the present, as he felt the warmth of his daughter's presence, this somewhat familiar woman smiling back at him. Dad took a deep breath as he reflected on the singing birds. He whistled, and I returned the tune. Yes, this was a good day, among the best we had ever known.

"Because I have a name,
gratitude turns everything into enough."

Portraits

Reaching out hands of support
and waving their portraits high.

Believe me when I say, I see the writing on the wall. This thief, the one who has stolen so much already, does not want you to hear it. The disease which has already stripped your loved one, and stripped you as well if he hasn't completely wiped you out, does not want you to be comforted. There is an urgency in this message which I do not pretend to understand.

I clearly see we are being attacked. The countless millions of us who walk beside the forty-four million folks in the world who live with Alzheimer's disease alone-and that is yesterday's statistic. Last year's best guess. There isn't even a statistic on us, the feet who walk beside them and are impacted right along with them. It is predicted that by 2025, less than a decade from now, over seven million of us, in the United States alone, will develop this disease.

I don't know about you, but I am still trying to wrap my head around five million. By 2050, when I will have just fifteen years left to prepare my centenarian wardrobe, it is projected that almost fourteen million people, in the

United States alone, will have the specific form of dementia known as Alzheimer's disease, barring medical breakthroughs to prevent or cure the disease. We only thought today's statistics were staggering.

This is of epidemic proportions. There is an urgency in this message and I need help spreading it. I phoned and emailed and texted my prayer warriors this morning, knowing I need help. This message needs to be told and it is imperative my voice be strong. Tears fill my eyes as I realize, once again, how much we have lost, how cruel this thief has been to us. Why did this disease have to strike my family, my friends, the family members of those I know and love? Why did it have to strike yours, my companions on this journey who I have yet to meet?

One of my husband's friends cared for his wife during her nine-year battle with Alzheimer's disease. The rest of his life will be spent paying the debt of her staggering medical costs. Another dear couple I recently met attends every lecture they can to learn as much as possible about this disease. He was recently diagnosed and spends hours a day at the gym to keep himself as active as possible in an attempt to stall the progression of this thief.

We do not have to imagine our most valued possessions have been stolen. It is painfully obvious and quite upsetting. Our hands are reaching out to someone we trust in desperate search of assistance. We need comfort, we need help, and we need it now. It is imperative this assailant be apprehended before he steals anything else, attempts to ruin any more lives.

We have but a vague recollection of what life used to be before this painful disease ripped us apart. Through visible distress, we acknowledge we have been robbed. There is not a soul who can deny it really happened. We are no longer hiding our portraits in the shadows. They are being brought into the light for all to see. We are raising them up and waving them in the air to announce to all: *We need some help!*

I did not fully understand it at the time, but I now understand that my tears were prayers. I was pouring out of these prayers for the millions upon millions of folks with invisible footprints who will be facing this disease very soon if we do not start fighting. They were prayers for the over four million individuals who silently face this walk every single day right now. They were intensely powerful cries to God. I was praying.

Help them!

It is presently costing $250 a day to keep my father in motion, and that is after we have dramatically cut expenses. We no longer have round the clock private care and Hospice has stepped in, thankfully. Don't get me wrong, I am not complaining. I would do anything to keep him going but after almost twelve years of these expenses, it is getting pretty tough.

Hospice has not only taken our hand to guide us through the next steps, they also provide all of Dad's medical supplies, including his shower chair, walker, and wheelchair. A Hospice nurse comes to give Dad a shower on Wednesdays, Tammy's day off, and brings Depends, wipes, bed pads, and anything else that is needed. When Hospice staff asked what size Depends my father wore I said, "You provide those for us?" She smiled. "Of course!" I cried. They were going to help us. Really step in and take some of this load. *I will help you!*

When I saw the message from my financial advisor, "My mom has Alzheimer's. It hurts me to see it." The message broke my heart. "Oh, wow!" I said. I had several of his mother's recipes in my collection. She even called me one year before Thanksgiving, knowing he had shared her cranberry salad recipe with me. She wanted to make sure I had her tips. (To insure I would not mess up her signature dish, I'm sure.) It has been our family's holiday staple ever since. I knew Joy moved to Assisted Living a few years ago and he even mentioned in passing a couple times he was concerned about her memory.

"I am so sorry. I was afraid that she might. When was she diagnosed?" I asked. I read his reply and it sent an urgency through my very core. "Well, what else could it be?" After explaining there were many causes, such as a UTI or medications that can cause short term memory loss that is reversible, I said, "Get her a diagnosis!

I have taken my portrait, the little girl my mother treasured, out of the closet. No longer will we hide our portraits. We have a story to tell! I received the proofs last night from the back cover photo shoot. The first picture is a precious photo of my dad. It is my portrait to show the world this man who is enduring so much because of this disease.

"Because I have a name, I believe God hears my prayers."

The Lighthouse

Learning to follow the unchanging light which forever guides our way.

I am on a mission and I can only hope I have presented the message loud and clearly. If I must shout it from the rooftops, let me tell you again:

Thank you for loving your loved one,
even on their most unlovable days.
They love you too.

One of the trademark signs of dementia is the absence in the eyes of those affected. They lack focus and many times, especially in the later stages of this disease, appear to be totally emotionless. Let me assure you, beyond the cloudy storms of dementia, there is a bright light shining within. Find your stone bench and sit with them in silence. Hold their hand and look, deep into the heart of their soul, just beyond their eyes, sick with heartache. You will find it. I promise you will.

I have been asked often over the years how I have walked this difficult road and survived. When I share my family's story, inevitably, I am implored to disclose my secret. With intensity resembling mine when I sought Aunt Lennie's century old tips, they ask, "Where has this fortitude come?" They want to know how I have been able to walk through the raging waters of this disease and emerge, not just a survivor, but stronger. I have only one answer because, if the truth be known, I am as weak and scared as they come.

If the years ahead had been displayed before me the day my father was diagnosed, I would have run the other way and never stopped. He was my lifeline; the strength I was counting on to walk with me through Mom's disease. Don't get me wrong, I love my parents and would have done absolutely anything for them. I believe this was proven the day I chose not to abandon them in the deli as the ugly folks sat in judgement.

But hear me when I say if I had known, truly understood, all the difficult decisions and impossible trials we would face, I would have been convinced I could not handle them on my own-and I would have been right. It was only because of my ability to focus on the obstacles of the day I was facing that I survived. Only due to being centered on living in the present moment without fearing the next, or regretting the past, that the waves of this terrible disease did not overwhelm me.

Please do not misunderstand me, there were many, many times I felt I was drowning. Difficult decisions to be made, moves to be faced, heartbreaking issues involving my parents' care to be endured, which violently tugged me underwater until I could not breath, then flung me to the shore, gasping for air.

I have become acutely aware of the feelings we suppress as caregivers. Honestly, we do not have time to feel, there is too much to do, and if we are not doing, we are worrying. Believe me when I say my husband and I have done our fair share of worrying lately. The expenses of this disease are astronomical. The mainstay of our income has plummeted, sinking in the abyss, right along with oil and gas prices.

Anyone who is walking this road knows what I mean when I say, no matter how brilliantly we plan for the expenses of this disease, in the end most of us are living on a prayer and a song. So even though there are many other things I need to be doing right now, I know there is absolutely nothing more important than reaching out to you and encouraging you to pick up your foot and walk the next step. Our loved ones are traveling right on down this road, whether we like it or not, and we can all agree we do not like it, not one bit.

Yet we keep walking. Although, if we are honest, we seldom feel worthy. We place the value of who we are on where we have been, and we don't have to glance too far over our shoulder to see the mistakes we have made. I have often thought: surely there are others who could have made better, more informed decisions for my parents' care. But the fact is, others were not chosen to be their daughter. It was me, The Big Surprise, who was called to walk this road. My sometimes unorthodox decisions have been put on display within the pages of this book to prove to the most doubtful among you: You can do this.

My parents were extremely private people and I wrestled with sharing their most personal moments. When my brother was murdered, I wrote in an attempt to make sense of the tragedy in my mind. Of course, this was not possible, to make sense of it, but writing was healing for me nonetheless. I shared some of these thoughts with my mom and she was horrified to read the horrible truth, displayed so naked and vulnerable. This disease is just that, a horrible truth, exposing its innocent, vulnerable victims.

So when I began to write, I had to wonder if Mom would have said, "Judith Ann, please don't expose us like this!

Don't let people see our shameful disease!" I thought this in my mind. However, in my heart, I knew it was not their fault. Their struggles, our challenges, had the potential to help someone else make sense of it all. At least some of it. I do know this, I can call to you from across the raging waters as I cling to the next jagged rock and say, "You can do it! It will be okay. We will work it out!" Rex taught us this. My parents would want you to know it too. Their story is shared so that you might believe.

Ultimately, I concluded my family's experiences have the potential to help others. If just one person can learn from my mistakes, just one insight be gleaned from the trials we faced, it will be worth the effort I have invested. If the successes I have stumbled on help others, then my decision to share our story was not in vain. My husband said this fervently and often: "If just one person hears your story, one family is encouraged, then it will all be worth it."

This was never about me. It was about you. **IT IS ABOUT THEM!** The message of hope, of love, of the light that will guide you through this darkest storm is what all of these words that have poured out of me and found their way onto the pages of this book are about.

There is something I need to share with you.
My final chapter, The Lighthouse, is a testimony:
how God carried me through this tragedy.
Without this, nothing else would have occurred as it did.
Without acknowledging Him, this book means nothing.

As it turns out, our footprints are invisible too. Jesus has been carrying us all along. In the end, this truth is all that matters.

I pray that your hearts will be flooded with light
so that you can understand the confident hope
He has given to those He called.
Ephesians 1:18

"Because I have a name, I will proclaim Your goodness for the rest of my life."

The Scrapbook

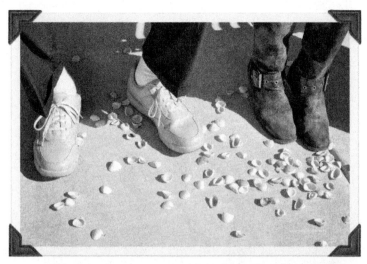

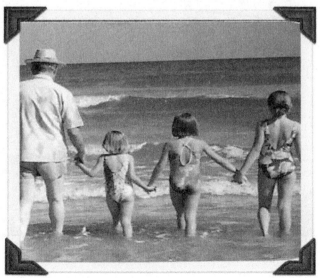

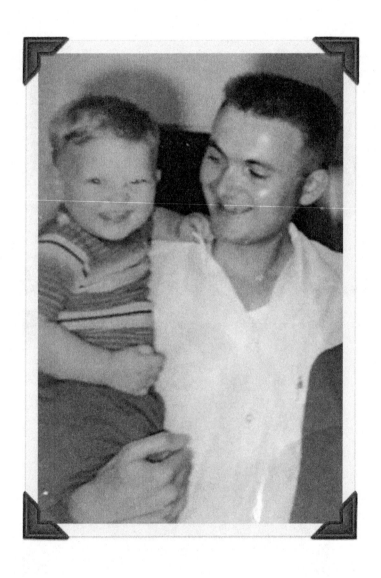

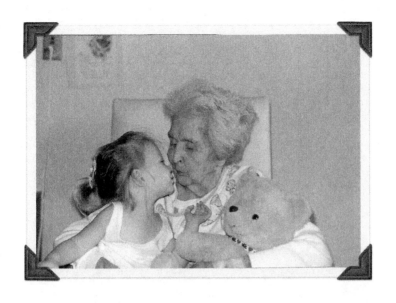

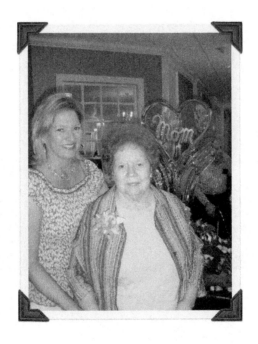

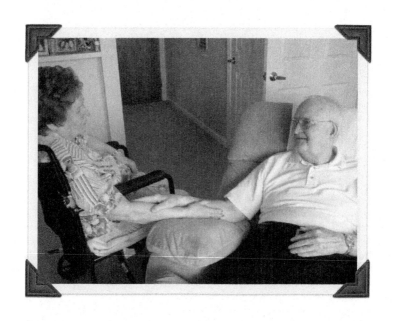

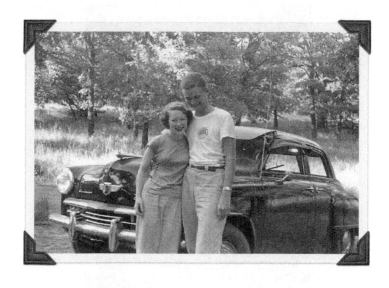

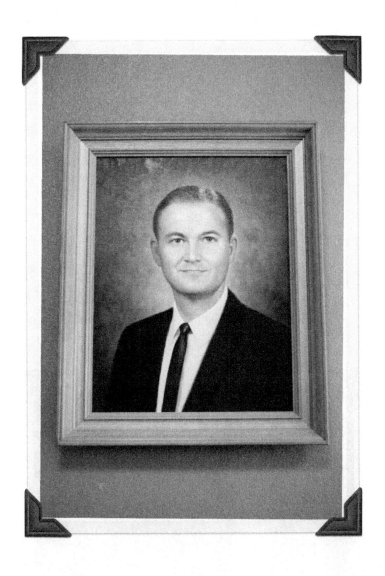

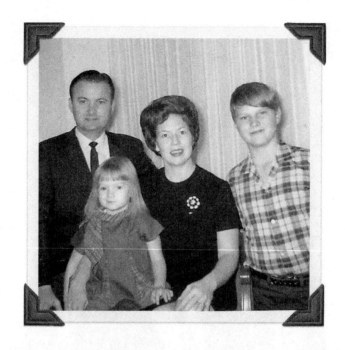

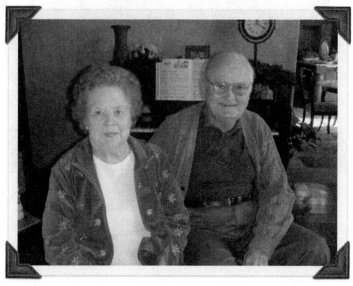

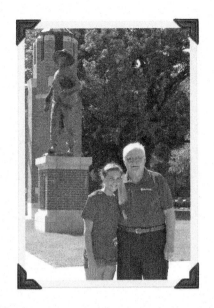

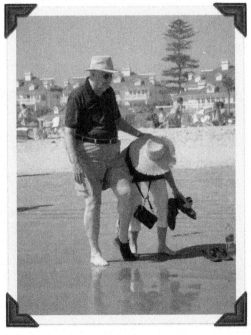

313

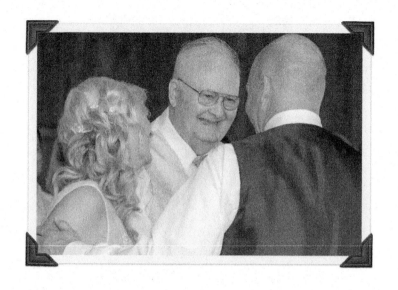

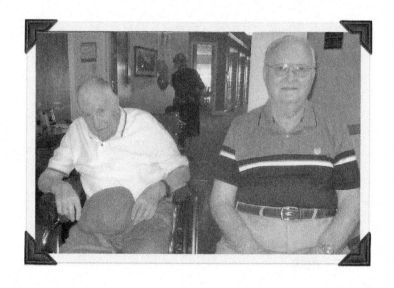

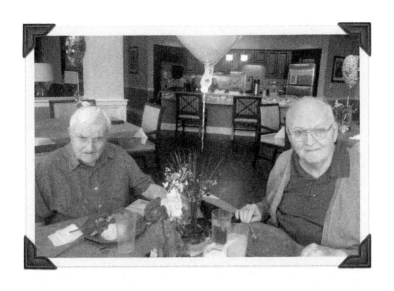

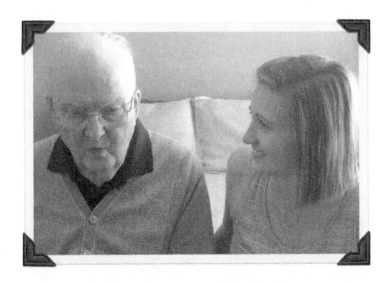

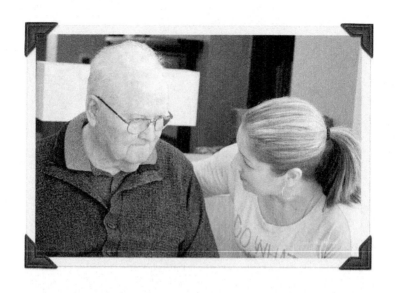

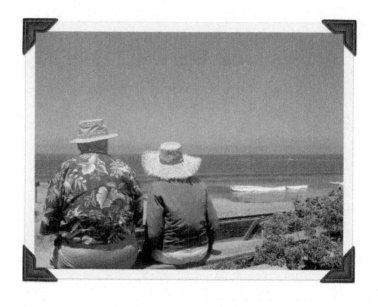

316

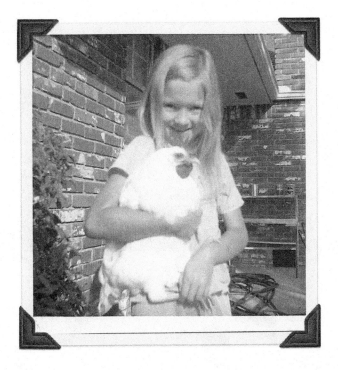

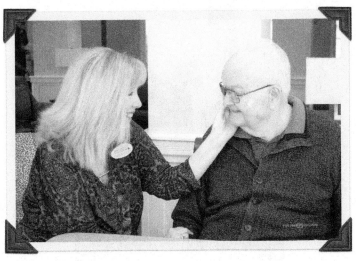

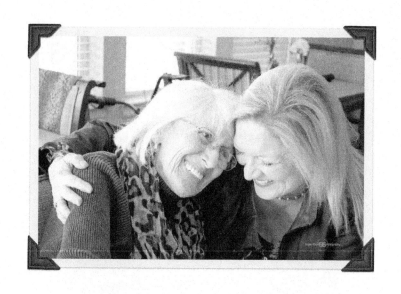

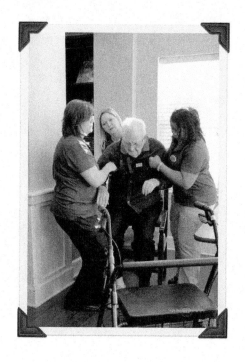

318

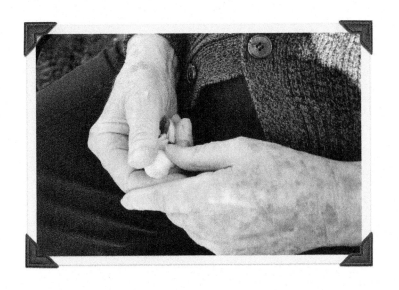

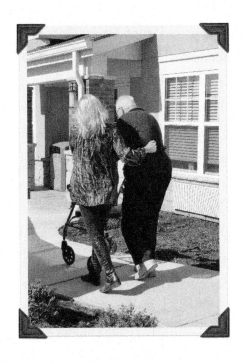

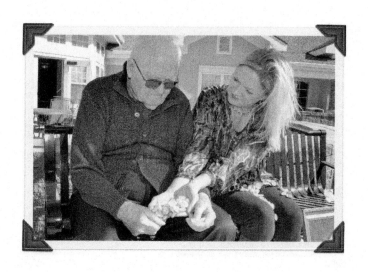

Through the process of working on this project,
I have learned much about life and love.
Most significantly, I am now acutely aware how much
these beautiful folks have to offer us-
much more than even I realized.
We may hold the treasured memories,
but they possess the keys to unlock them.
Eventually, they will arrive at a place of contentment
where grudges are held no longer,
laughter is abundant, and an awareness
of the needs of others is refined.
I have discovered in the process of attempting
to help them,
My life has been profoundly touched and changed
for the better.

Common Causes and Characteristics of Dementia
Alzheimer's Association 2015
Alzheimer's Disease Facts and Figures Report

Alzheimer's disease

Most common cause of dementia; accounts for an estimated 60-80 percent of cases. About half of these cases involve solely Alzheimer's pathology; many have evidence of pathologic changes related to other dementias. This is called mixed dementia (see mixed dementia)

Difficulty remembering recent conversations, names or events is often an early clinical symptom; apathy and depression are also often early symptoms. Later symptoms include impaired communication, disorientation, confusion, poor judgment, behavior changes and, ultimately, difficulty speaking, swallowing, and walking.

Revised criteria and guidelines for diagnosing Alzheimer's were proposed and published in 2011. These recommend that Alzheimer's be considered a slowly progressive brain disease that begins well before clinical symptoms emerge.

The hallmark pathologies of Alzheimer's are the progressive accumulation of the protein fragment beta-amyloid (plaques) outside neurons in the brain and twisted strands of the protein tau (tangles) inside neurons. These changes are eventually accompanied by the damage and death of neurons.

Vascular dementia

Previously known as multi-infarct or post-stroke dementia, vascular dementia is less common as a sole cause of dementia than Alzheimer's, accounting for about 10 percent of dementia cases. However, it is very common in older individuals with dementia, with about 50 percent having pathologic evidence of vascular dementia (infarcts). In most cases, the infarcts coexist with Alzheimer's pathology. (see mixed dementia)

Impaired judgment or impaired ability to make decisions, plan or organize is more likely to be the initial symptom, as opposed to the memory loss often associated with the initial symptoms of Alzheimer's. Vascular dementia occurs most commonly from blood vessel blockage or damage leading to infarcts (strokes) or bleeding in the brain. The location, number, and size of the brain injuries determine whether dementia will result and how the individual's thinking and physical functioning will be affected.

In the past, evidence of vascular dementia was used to exclude a diagnosis of Alzheimer's (and vice versa). That practice is no longer considered consistent with the pathologic evidence, which shows that the brain changes of Alzheimer's and vascular dementia commonly coexist. When evidence of two or more causes of dementia are present at the same time, the individual is considered to have mixed dementia.

Dementia with Lewy bodies (DLB)

People with DLB have some of the symptoms common in Alzheimer's, but are more likely to have initial or early symptoms of sleep disturbances, well-formed visual hallucinations and slowness, gait imbalance, or other parkinsonian movement features. These features, as well as early visuospatial impairment, may occur in the absence of significant memory impairment.

Lewy bodies are abnormal aggregations (or clumps) of the protein alpha-synuclein that accumulate in neurons. When they develop in a part of the brain called the cortex, dementia can result. Alpha-synuclein also aggregates in the brains of people with Parkinson's disease (PD), in which it is accompanied by severe neuronal loss in a part of the brain called the substantia nigra. While people with DLB and PD both have Lewy bodies, the onset of the disease is marked by motor impairment in PD and cognitive impairment in DLB.

The brain changes of DLB alone can cause dementia. But very commonly brains with DLB have coexisting Alzheimer's pathology. In people with both DLB and Alzheimer's pathology, symptoms of both diseases may emerge and lead to some confusion in diagnosis. Vascular dementia can also coexist and contribute to the dementia. When evidence of more than one dementia is present, the individual is said to have mixed dementia. (see mixed dementia in this table).

Mixed dementia

Characterized by the hallmark abnormalities of more than one cause of dementia - most commonly Alzheimer's combined with vascular dementia, followed by Alzheimer's with DLB, and Alzheimer's with vascular dementia and DLB. Vascular dementia with DLB is much less common.

Recent studies suggest that mixed dementia is more common than previously recognized, with about half of those with dementia having pathologic evidence of more than one cause of dementia.

Parkinson's disease (PD) dementia

Problems with movement (slowness, rigidity, tremor, and changes in gait) are common symptoms of PD. In PD, alpha-synuclein aggregates appear in an area deep in the brain called the substantia nigra. The aggregates are thought to cause degeneration of the nerve cells that produce dopamine. The incidence of PD is about one-tenth that of Alzheimer's.

As PD progresses, it often results in dementia secondary to the accumulation of Lewy bodies in the cortex (similar to DLB) or the accumulation of beta-amyloid clumps and tau tangles (similar to Alzheimer's disease).

Creutzfeldt-Jakob disease

This very rare and rapidly fatal disorder impairs memory and coordination and causes behavior changes. Results from a misfolded protein (prion) that causes other proteins throughout the brain to misfold and malfunction.

May be hereditary (caused by a gene that runs in one's family), sporadic (unknown cause), or caused by a known prion infection. A specific form called variant Creutzfeldt-Jakob disease is believed to be caused by consumption of products from cattle affected by mad cow disease.

Normal pressure hydrocephalus

Symptoms include difficulty walking, memory loss, and inability to control urination. Accounts for less than 5 percent of dementia cases.

Caused by impaired reabsorption of cerebrospinal fluid and the consequent build-up of fluid in the brain, increasing pressure in the brain.

People with a history of brain hemorrhage (particularly subarchnoid hemorrhage) and meningitis are at increased risk. Can sometimes be corrected with surgical installation of a shunt in the brain to drain excess fluid.

Frontotemporal lobar degeneration (FTLD)

Includes dementias such as behavioral-variant FTLD, primary progressive aphasia, Pick's disease, corticobasal degeneration, and progressive supranuclear palsy.

Typical early symptoms include marked changes in personality and behavior and difficulty with producing or comprehending language. Unlike Alzheiimer's, memory is typically spared in the early stages of disease.

Nerve cells in the front (frontal lobe) and side regions (temporal lobes) of the brain are especially affected, and these regions become markedly atrophied (shrunken). In addition, the upper protein or the transactive response SNA-binding protein).

The brain changes of behavioral-variant FTLD may occur in those age 65 years and older, similar to Alzheimer's disease, but most people with this form of dementia develop symptoms at a younger age (at about age 60). In this younger age group, FTLD is the second most common degenerative dementia.

* For more information on these and other causes of dementia, visit alz.org/dementia

Helpful Resources

Alive Inside - http://www.alz.org/

Within a topic often epitomized by bleakness, isolation, and loss, this Sundance documentary uncovers inspiring and transformative occurrences of music therapy that gifts sufferers of dementia precious moments of clarity. In his first feature length documentary, filmmaker Michael Rossato-Bennett follows social worker Dan Cohen's methods of utilizing our primitive and ingrained responses to music, both cognitive and emotional, in an effort to maintain and invigorate his subjects' basic humanity.

The Alzheimer's Association - http://www.alz.org/

The leading voluntary health organization in Alzheimer's care, support, and research. Their website provides a wealth of information, resources, and news of upcoming events, training seminars, and support groups. https://www.alz.org/facts/downloads/facts_figures_2015.pdf

Alzheimer's Association Helpline - 24/7

Call 800-272-3900

Areawide Aging Agency - www.areawideaging.org

Caregiver Connection -

http://www.caregiverconnectionllc.com/

Founder, Paula Avery, insures help is available. Many people are thrust into a care giving situation not knowing who to call, who can help, or even when they should call for assistance. Caregiver Connection, LLC is the place to start. Through an in depth personal consultation you can sit down one- on-one with a professional to discuss your situation and get the guidance you need.

Dementia Instructor - http://dementiainstructor.com/

Melva Noakes brings nearly two decades of quality senior care to this website. Through her drive and dedication to serve individuals with Alzheimer's disease and other forms of dementia, she has voluntarily initiated and completed extensive training to provide care and training for those affected.

Music and Memory - musicandmemory.org

A non-profit organization that brings personalized music into the lives of the elderly or infirm through digital music technology, vastly improving quality of life. Train nursing home staff and other elder care professionals, as well as family caregivers, how to create and provide personalized playlists using iPods and related digital audio systems that enable those struggling with Alzheimer's, dementia and other cognitive and physical challenges to reconnect with the world through music-triggered memories.

Lost Chord - www.lost-chord.org.uk

An innovative charity in the UK dedicated to improving the quality of life and well-being of those suffering with dementia using interactive musical stimuli to increase their general awareness and self esteem.

Paro Robotic Seals - parorobotsus.com

Interactive therapy robots developed by Dr. Takanori Shibata, a Japanese scientist. These interactive robotic animals are designed to reduce depression and anxiety in dementia patients. Now available in the U.S., Dr. Sandra Petersen, of the University of Texas at Tyler is conducting research and doctors are beginning to prescribe sessions with these adorable seals in place of medications.

Purple Elephant - https://thepurpleelephant.org/

A nonprofit organization that is changing the way young people think about Alzheimer's disease on a global scale. Commitment and passion to empower young people and inspire communities to be agents of change. This organization works to provide in-home caregiving relief to individuals and families whose lives have been impacted while caring for a loved one with Alzheimer's. Their members, "The Purple Tribe" are active in the community, standing in unity as awareness of Alzheimer's disease is raised. The ultimate goal is a world where Alzheimer's is but a distant memory.

Respite Care -

http://www.careteamhc.com/respite-voucher-program/
Provides financial assistance to family caregivers in the form of vouchers that can be used to pay for respite care so the caregiver can take a break. Look for similar programs in your area.

Sunbeam Family Services -
http://sunbeamfamilyservices.org
Provides people of all ages with help, hope, and the opportunity to
succeed. Provides volunteers throughout the US as senior companions
to offer respite to their caregivers free of charge. Also is a source for
Care Trak, a bracelet that works as an emergency locator transmitter.
This tracker is designed for individuals who are prone to wandering.
Look for similar programs in your area.

Teepa Snow - http://teepasnow.com/
Care strategies & techniques integrating what is known about brain
function and changes that happen with dementing conditions with
therapeutic approaches. Teepa teaches about the value of connection
when primary verbal communication and interaction abilities are
altered. Her teaching style is extraordinarily unique in that she is able to
accurately demonstrate and model for her students and audience the
struggle and challenges dementia creates for all parties involved.

TrialMatch - trialmatch.alz.org/find-clinical-trials
Alzheimer's Association TrialMatch is a free, easy-to-use clinical
studies matching service that connects individuals with Alzheimer's,
caregivers, healthy volunteers and physicians with current studies. Our
continuously updated database of Alzheimer's clinical trials includes
more than 260 promising clinical studies being conducted at over 700
trials sites across the country.

U.S. Department of Veterans Affairs -
www.benefits.va.gov/benefits/
The Department of Veterans Affairs (VA) will provide benefits and
services that address a variety of issues, including health risks and
financial challenges, through VA benefits and services for Veterans and
their dependents. Additionally, special consideration is now being
given to those suffering with Parkinson's disease.

Book Resources For Caregivers

1. **Creating Moments of Joy for the Person with Alzheimer's or Dementia** Jun 2000 by Jolene Brackey. Alzheimer's & Dementia Books for Caregivers. Caregivers need comfort too and few people know this fact better than those caring for someone with Alzheimer's.

2. **Caregiver's Reprieve 3. The 36-Hour Day: A Family Guide to Caring for People With Alzheimer's Disease, Other Dementias, and Memory Loss in Later Life** *by Nancy L. Mace and Peter V. Rabins. 4th ed. Baltimore: Johns Hopkins University Press, 2006* Considered the "Bible" for families caring for a loved one with AD, this book features practical advice and plenty of examples covering all aspects of care, including emotional issues of caring, financial details, and day-to-day coping with dementia behaviors. Also includes information about nursing homes and other types of residential living.

3. **Mayo Clinic Guide to Alzheimer's Disease: The Essential Resource for Treatment, Coping and Caregiving** *by Ronald Petersen, ed. Rochester, MN: Mayo Clinic Health Solutions, 2006* If you're looking for a book that explains how Alzheimer's and other types of dementia affect the brain, but without confusing medical jargon, this concise guide outlines how the brain works, what constitutes healthy aging, signs and symptoms of Alzheimer's, as well as recent developments in diagnosis and treatment. It also includes a caregiver action plan with tips on medication administration, behavior management, home safety, and more.

4. **The Alzheimer's Action Plan: The Experts' Guide to the Best Diagnosis and Treatment for Memory Problems** *by P. Murali Doraiswamy; Lisa Gwyther. New York: St. Martin's Press, 2008* Families and health professionals alike will find a wealth of advice in this book, which was co- written by a social worker and a physician who is expert in AD and dementia. In addition to providing a guide to diagnosis and treatment methods, it outlines coping strategies for life after diagnosis, including what to expect from different stages of the disease and how to participate in clinical trials.

5. **Alzheimer's Early Stages: First Steps for Family, Friends and Caregivers** *by Daniel Kuhn, MSW, and David A. Bennett, MD. 2nd ed. Alameda, CA: Hunter House Publishers, 2003* This book is unique in its focus on the early stages of Alzheimer's and how families can better understand and cope with its effects as their loved one begins to experience cognitive and behavioral changes. Beyond practical coping advice, it provides suggestions on how to handle caregiver stress, an extensive list of resources, and a section consisting of first-person accounts by caregivers and family members who have faced similar situations.

6. **The Forgetting. Alzheimer's: Portrait of an Epidemic** *by David Shenk. New York: Random House, Inc., 2003* Shenk is a journalist and NPR commentator who has written more than just a book about AD, but a moving exploration of the nature of memory and the history of the disease from its discovery to the present. He discusses the role of scientists, caregivers, and policymakers in the treatment history of the disease, giving examples of well-known personages who suffered from Alzheimer's. The National Institute on Aging calls

it "a readable, accessible description of the history of AD, research, and the human impact of the disease."

7. **Alzheimer's Disease: Unraveling the Mystery** *National Institutes of Health, 2008.* This free NIH publication can be downloaded in PDF format or ordered as a print copy from the National Institute on Aging's website. It takes a closer look at the healthy aging brain in comparison to the brain with Alzheimer's, covers the latest information from the frontlines of diagnostic and treatment research, and talks about the need to improve caregiver support across a broad spectrum, especially for family caregivers.

8. **Understanding difficult behaviors: some practical suggestions for coping with Alzheimer's disease and related illnesses** *A. Robinson, B. Spencer, and L. White. Eastern Michigan University, Ypsilanti, MI: 2007* According to the Alzheimer's Association, "This resource receives high praise for its format, specific hard-to-find information, and practical steps to take when faced with a variety of behaviors." It helps families and caregivers understand why challenging behaviors occur, how to communicate, and how to cope. It's also recommended by the Family Caregiver Alliance and the NC Department of Health and Human Services.

9. **Activities to Do with Your Parent Who Has Alzheimer's Dementia** *by Judith Levy, EdM, OTR. CreateSpace Independent Publishing Platform, 2014* This book offers user-friendly activities and a means to objectively assess if the activities helped or need to be adapted. This resource enables consistency and communication between caregivers which benefits the loved one.

10. **The 36-Hour Day: A Family Guide to Caring for People With Alzheimer's Disease, Other Dementias, and Memory Loss in Later Life** *by Nancy L. Mace and Peter V. Rabins. 4th ed. Baltimore: Johns Hopkins University Press, 2006* Considered the "Bible" for families caring for a loved one with AD, this book features practical advice and plenty of examples covering all aspects of care, including emotional issues of caring, financial details, and day-to-day coping with dementia behaviors. Also includes information about nursing homes and other types of residential living.

Resource: Sarah J. Stevenson,
http://www.sarahjamilastevenson.com

Acknowledgements

My deepest gratitude to those providing physical and medical care for my parents over the past 12 years. It took us all. I could not have done this without you. Thank you.

The original four: Karen, Bonita, Mila, Tammy

Abena	Carolyn	Debi
Alsace	Cathy	Debra
Amal	Chad	DeeDee
Andy	Charlie B.	Delica
Angie	Charlie F.	Diagnostic
Ann	Charmaine	Staff
Antoinette	Cherie	Dillon
Barbara	Cherie R.	Don
Bea	Cheryl	Donita
Benice	Chris	Donna
Becky	Cinthia	Donna J.
Bill	Clayborn	Doug
Bill B.	Corri	Emma
Bill H.	Crystal	Ethyl
Billie	Cynthia	Feeschell
Billy	Dale	Fountains Staff
Bobby	Dan	Greg
Bonnie	Dani	Home Health
Brenda	Danny	Staff
Britta	Dave	Ian
Bruce	David	Jacques
Carola	Debbie	Jaime

Jamari

Jennifer

Jerrod

Jessica

Jim

Joann

Josh

Judy

June

Julie

Kathy

Kay

Kendra

Kenny

Kevyn

Kierra

Kim

Kim

Kip

Kristen

Kristen D.

Kwame

Lance

Larry

LaTeva

Lee

Leese

Leslie

Linda

Lisa

Lois

Lonnie

Lorna

Luz

Marcus

Marian

Melisha

Melva

Mercy Hospital
Staff

Michelle

Mickey

Monika

Morgan

Nakia

Nancy

Nelson

Neoma

Norma

Pam

Patty

Paula

Physical
Therapy Staff

Ranessa

Rose

Rex

Sally

Sandra

Sara

Scott

Shameka

Sharon

Sierra

Skilled Nursing
Staff

Steph

Steve

Susan

Susan C.

Sylvia

Terri

Tracy

Ulf

———————

The following
doctors & staff:

Dr. Crain

Dr. Dasharathy

Dr. Little

Dr. Ross

Dr. Scott

Dr. Shaw

Dr. Sparkes

Dr. Wasemiller-
Smith

Dr. Woods

Even When It Hurts by Joel Houston

Following the journey of the song through the first four times
we ever played it live, from studio to arena—
There is a parallel to be found within the narrative of seasons and days,
the constant-unpredictability of life, and the unchanging, unfailing nature of God
and His faithfulness — and what singing His praises unlocks in us.

In this journey, the song serves as the constant and honest-confession within us,
as the environment and atmosphere changes like the seasons come-and-go around us. Even When it Hurts is a Praise Song —
This is the kind written to sound its loudest in the cold-lonely-silence of the darkest night, or the heart-drenched-desperation of the heaviest of tears.

It's a song that finds its voice in the moments and seasons,
where to all common sense and logic, to sing,
and be thankful for anything at all,
let alone sing a song of praise to God,
makes no sense at all -

when the fight seems lost and all strength gone with it -
when it's hard to even find the words - louder then,
this is that kind of praise song.

CPSIA information can be obtained
at www.ICGtesting.com
Printed in the USA
LVOW04s2336280316

481165LV00032B/852/P